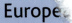

European ncology

Handbook of Oncological Emergencies

Edited by

Paris A. Kosmidis
Athens, Greece

Dirk Schrijvers
Antwerp, Belgium

Fabrice André
Villejuif, France

Sylvie Rottey
Ghent, Belgium

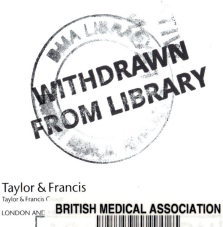

Taylor & Francis
Taylor & Francis G

LONDON AND

© 2005 Taylor & Francis, an imprint of the Taylor & Francis Group

First published in the United Kingdom in 2005
by Taylor & Francis, an imprint of the Taylor & Francis Group, 2 Park Square, Milton Park, Abingdon, Oxon, OX14 4RN

Tel.:   +44 (0) 20 7017 6000
Fax.:   +44 (0) 20 7017 6699
E-mail: info.medicine@tandf.co.uk
Website: http://www.tandf.co.uk/medicine

A CIP record for this book is available from the British Library.

Library of Congress Cataloging-in-Publication Data

Data available on application

ISBN 1 84184 523 X

Distributed in North and South America by

Taylor & Francis
2000 NW Corporate Blvd
Boca Raton, FL 33431, USA

Within Continental USA
Tel.: 800 272 7737; Fax.: 800 374 3401
Outside Continental USA
Tel.: 561 994 0555; Fax.: 561 361 6018
E-mail: orders@crcpress.com

Distributed in the rest of the world by
Thomson Publishing Services
Cheriton House
North Way
Andover, Hampshire SP10 5BE, UK
Tel.: +44 (0)1264 332424
E-mail: salesorder.tandf@thomsonpublishingservices.co.uk

Composition by Creative, Scotland

Printed and bound in Italy by Printer Trento

This publication has been supported by an unrestricted educational grant from
Ortho Biotech, the Biopharmaceutical Division of Janssen-Cilag

Contents

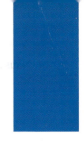

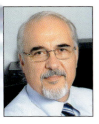

Paris A. Kosmidis, MD
Hygeia Hospital in Athens, Greece

President of the European Society for Medical
Oncology

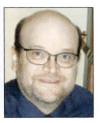

Prof. Dirk Schrijvers, MD, PhD
*Antwerp Oncological Centre, ZNA Middelheim, Antwerp,
Belgium*

Chairman of the European Society for Medical
Oncology Educational Committee

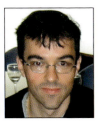

Fabrice André, MD, PhD
Institute Gustave Roussy, Villejuif, France

Steering Committee Chairman of the European Society
for Medical Oncology Young Medical Oncologists
Working Group

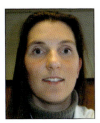

Sylvie Rottey, MD
University Hospital of Ghent, Belgium

Steering Committee Member of the European Society
for Medical Oncology Young Medical Oncologists
Working Group

Preface

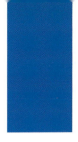

It is with great pleasure that I introduce this *Handbook of Oncological Emergencies*, a publication initiated by the European Society for Medical Oncology's (ESMO) Young Medical Oncologists Working Group.

Our Society has gathered together promising young colleagues in an effort to effectively prepare and uniformly train them to be future oncology leaders. ESMO has invested both time and resources in a career development program for this group through fellowships, educational training, special congress sessions and symposia, and masterclasses.

Providing oncologists with guidelines on emergency treatments through this handbook represents only one portion of our Society's comprehensive program to invest in the future of oncology in Europe.

The chapters have been written by distinguished young medical oncologists and supervised by senior colleagues, whom I sincerely thank. I also wish to express my deep gratitude to my co-editors, Prof. Dirk Schrijvers, Dr. Fabrice André and Dr Sylvie Rottey for their hard work and excellent collaboration, and to Taylor & Francis, the publisher of this ESMO handbook. And I add very special thanks to Ortho Biotech for their generous support of this publication through an unrestricted educational grant.

It is my sincere hope that this handbook will be of use and service to you.

Paris A. Kosmidis
ESMO President

Cardiac complications of cancer and anticancer treatment

G de Castro Jr, M Hatsue
Honda Federico Hospital das Clínicas, Brazil

Malignant pericardial effusion and cardiac tamponade

Etiology

Involvement of the pericardium is most frequently observed in patients with advanced lung and breast cancer, leukemia, lymphomas and malignant melanoma. The onset of symptoms may be gradual or rapid, depending on the rate of fluid accumulation. As fluid accumulates, the subsequent increase in intrapericardial pressure affects the diastolic filling of the heart, leading to a restrictive cardiac output reduction.

Chemotherapy-related effusions are rare but may be seen with busulfan, cytarabine or tretinoin.

Differential diagnosis

Differential diagnosis includes superior vena cava syndrome, radiation pericarditis, myocardial infarction, infections (bacterial, viral, fungal), connective tissue disorders, myxedema, trauma, uremia and serum hypoalbuminemia.

Evaluation of pericardial effusion and cardiac tamponade

- Pericardial effusions may be frequently asymptomatic. Symptoms associated with pericardium involvement are dyspnea, chest pain, cough, palpitations, orthopnea, fatigue and weakness, anxiety and confusion, fever, hiccups, oliguria and edema.
- Physical signs that may be noted on presentation are tachycardia, decreased heart sounds, neck vein distension, peripheral edema and pericardial friction rubs.
- As cardiac tamponade develops, hypotension, arrhythmia and elevation of the central venous pressure can be observed. A hallmark, when present, is

- pulsus paradoxus, defined as an inspiratory decrease of more than 10 mmHg in the systolic pressure. Patients may develop a low-output shock.
- Two-dimensional echocardiography is considered the standard method for diagnosing pericardial effusion. It can detect circumferential and loculated pericardial effusions and can reveal right atrial and right ventricular collapse during diastole, which strongly suggest pericardial tamponade.
- The initial evaluation of the patient usually includes a chest radiograph, which may provide evidence of an enlarged cardiac silhouette. However, a very small effusion or a rapidly accumulating effusion with normal chest radiography is not uncommon.
- Electrocardiogram (ECG) is rarely useful but low-voltage complexes and electrical alternans have been described as suggestive for pericardial effusion.
- A computed tomography (CT) scan is an alternative in patients in whom echocardiography cannot be used to identify fluid in the pericardial sac, such as in obese patients or in the presence of chronic obstructive pulmonary disease.
- Cardiac catheterization confirms the presence of pericardial tamponade and helps in the quantitation of hemodynamic compromise.
- Pericardiocentesis establishes the etiology of the effusion and should be performed promptly if the patient presents with signs of cardiac tamponade. Biochemical, cytologic and microbiological analyses of the pericardial fluid are mandatory.
- Pericardial biopsy may be necessary, but the diagnostic yield is less than the cytologic examination. Confirming the malignant nature of the pericardial effusion depends on the recognition of malignant cells at the cytologic examination or documentation of a pericardial metastasis at the biopsy.

Treatment

Treatment depends on the underlying etiology and symptom progression.

In patients with no or minimal symptoms without hemodynamic implications, systemic management is warranted, especially in patients with chemosensitive cancers (lymphomas, leukemias, small cell lung cancer and breast cancer). Radiotherapy may be indicated for pericardial effusion associated with lymphomas, breast and lung cancers. The extension of pericardial effusion and response to therapy may be followed by echocardiograms.

For patients with tamponade, immediate pericardiocentesis is lifesaving and is mandatory.

- In case of mild hypotension, a rapid intravenous infusion of normal saline or Ringer's lactate may increase the right ventricular filling pressure above the pericardial pressure and thereby improve momentarily the cardiac output.
- Pericardiocentesis is performed using a small-gauge spinal needle (20–22 gauge) connected to the V lead of an ECG, through a subxiphoid approach, with echocardiography guidance. The needle is introduced under local anesthesia and is directed from the subxiphoid skin entry site to the apex of the left shoulder. If the epicardial surface is touched, ST-segment elevation and premature ventricular contractions are seen. Once the pericardial space is entered, a guidewire is introduced, the needle is removed, and a catheter inserted over the guidewire. The catheter may be left in place for drainage and instillation of sclerosing agents. Malignant pericardial fluid is usually exudative and often hemorrhagic. The catheter may be left in place until the amount of drained fluid had dropped to less than 75–100 ml per day.
- Systolic dysfunction may follow the relief of tamponade, with spontaneous recovery in 2 weeks.
- In patients in whom there is no systemic therapy to control the pericardial effusion, local measures should be considered based on the type and extension of the disease, previous treatments, performance status and overall prognosis:
  - subxiphoid pericardiostomy/pericardial window may be performed, especially for those patients with a longer life expectancy. It also provides samples for analysis
  - pericardiostomy with intrapericardial instillation of sclerosing agents (more commonly with bleomycin and doxycycline).
- Recurrent effusions can be approached by:
  - transthoracic pleuropericardial window
  - pericardioperitoneal shunt.
- Pericardiectomy is usually reserved for patients with post-irradiation pericarditis.
- Acute radiation-induced pericarditis should be managed conservatively with non-steroidal anti-inflammatory drugs or corticosteroids.

Cardiomyopathy and congestive heart failure (CHF)

Etiology

Chemotherapy regimens with anthracycline antibiotics, such as doxorubicin, epirubicin, daunorubicin and idarubicin, are the most frequent causes of congestive heart failure (CHF). The biventricular CHF, as a consequence of anthracycline-induced cardiomyopathy (AIC), is usually cumulative and dose-related.

Mitoxantrone, cyclophosphamide, ifosfamide (the last two alkylating agents when used in high-dose regimens), paclitaxel (specially in combination with anthracyclines), mitomycin C (after anthracyclines), interleukin-2, alfa-interferon and trastuzumab are other drugs associated with cardiomyopathy.

The incidence of CHF as a result of doxorubicin cardiotoxicity is estimated as varying from 7% to 15% in patients receiving cumulative doses higher than 450–500 mg/m^2. Higher doses are thought to raise CHF incidence more steeply. However, lower cumulative doses do not guarantee CHF will not occur. Over the age of 70 years old, an increased risk of AIC needs to be considered in association with previous exposure to ionizing radiation to the chest, other cardiac conditions such as pre-existing active CHF and ischemia or hypertension, or prior exposure to anthracyclines.

Evaluation

- Patients with AIC may have a subacute presentation with mild symptoms and few clinical signs of CHF as tachycardia, dyspnea, decreased exercise tolerance and pulmonary and circulatory congestion.
- Doppler echocardiography is a useful method to evaluate the baseline cardiac volumes and left ventricular ejection fraction (LVEF) and for the follow-up during treatment.
- Gated radionuclide scan with multiple acquisitions (MUGA scan) is also used to evaluate AIC. Patients treated with doxorubicin should be submitted to an evaluation of the LVEF at baseline, 300 mg/m^2 and 450 mg/m^2 cumulative doses, and each 100 mg/m^2 thereafter. Decrease in LVEF from 10 to 20% in absolute value or to less than 45% warrants discontinuation of therapy.
- Endomyocardial biopsies obtained by heart catheterization and evaluated by routine histologic and electron-microscopic examination can reveal a continuum of changes induced by anthracyclines, relatively specific, and these changes appear to parallel the clinical and scan alterations.

Prevention and treatment

■ AIC can be prevented by changing the intravenous (IV) bolus schedule (usually used with a 21-day interval) to 3- to 4-day continuous infusion or weekly schedules, and empirically limiting cumulative doses of doxorubicin to 450–500 mg/m^2. Although epirubicin has a better profile of cardiac toxicity than doxorubicin, the risk of CHF increases significantly with cumulative doses over 900 mg/m^2 in patients with no previous anthracycline exposure.

■ Dexrazoxane IV, at 10:1 dexrazoxane:doxorubicin ratio might be given 30 minutes before doxorubicin in order to prevent and/or to reduce the chance of AIC in women with metastatic breast cancer, who have been previously exposed to a total cumulative dose of doxorubicin 300 mg/m^2 or higher and who might still benefit from additional anthracycline treatment. It is not recommended for patients starting doxorubicin-based therapy or in adjuvant setting.

■ There is currently no therapy that can reverse the AIC:
  – cardiotoxic regimens must be stopped and fluid and sodium restriction must be prescribed
  – diuretics and digoxin can offer some relief for the congestive states
  – clinical improvement can result from afterload reduction with angiotensin-converting enzyme inhibitors, carvedilol and spironolactone
  – patients who have been refractory to treatment and are malignancy-free can be considered as candidates for cardiac transplantation.

Myocardial ischemia

Etiology

The most common drug used in the treatment of cancer associated with myocardial ischemia is 5-fluorouracil, especially when used in continuous infusion (1–4.5% incidence) and in combination with cisplatin.

Radiation therapy to the chest is also implicated as an initial cause and in the worsening of a pre-existing coronary artery disease.

Evaluation

■ Patients usually present with thoracic pain, similar to other coronary syndromes, but can also present with ventricular arrhythmias and cardiac arrest.

- ECG may evidence an ST-segment elevation and may be suggestive of myocardial infarction.
- Coronary angiography is usually consistent with coronary artery spasm.

Treatment

If ischemia occurs during 5-fluorouracil infusion, it must be immediately stopped and nitrates (IV nitroglycerin) and calcium channel blockers should be used to control the coronary artery spasm, even if they are ineffective in preventing the spasm. This manifestation is reversible. Controlled underlying ischemia should not be considered an absolute contraindication to further treatment with 5-fluorouracil.

Arrhythmias

Etiology

Arrhythmias can be related to coronary or myocardial disease secondary to cancer therapy or direct arrhythmogenic effects of therapy. Sinus tachycardia is commonly found in patients with anthracycline-induced cardiomyopathy, as well as other supra- and ventricular arrhythmias. Amsacrine infusion is associated with prolongation of the QT interval. Paclitaxel occasionally causes asymptomatic bradycardia.

Evaluation

Diagnosis is based on ECG changes.

Treatment

The drug involved must be withdrawn and the arrhythmia appropriately treated. Events that are not life-threatening may be managed conservatively, but whenever hemodynamic instability is imminent or life-threatening, active intervention according to advanced cardiac life-support protocols is mandatory (Table 1.1). Metabolic abnormalities should be corrected and other possibly arrythmogenic drugs should also be withdrawn.

Table 1.1 Treatment of arrhythmias

Arrhythmia	Treatment
Supraventricular tachycardia	β-blocker
	Verapamil
Atrial fibrillation	β-blocker
	Diltiazem
	Cardioversion
	Amiodarone IV in unstable patients
	Anticoagulation
Ventricular tachycardia (sustained)	Amiodarone IV
	Implantable defibrillation in selected patients

Further reading

Abeloff MD, Armitage JO, Lichter AS, Niederhuber JE: Clinical Oncology, 2nd edn. Philadelphia: Churchill Livingstone, 2000.

De Vita VT Jr, Hellman S, Rosenberg SA: Cancer: Principles and Practice of Oncology, 6th edn. Philadelphia: Lippincott-Raven, 2001.

Hancock EW: Neoplastic pericardial disease. Cardiol Clin 1990; 8: 673–82.

Keefe DL: Anthracycline-induced cardiomyopathy. Semin Oncol 2001; 28 (4 suppl 12): 2–7.

Schuchter LM, Hensley ML, Meropol NJ et al: 2002 update of recommendations for the use of chemotherapy and radiotherapy protectants: clinical practice guidelines of the American Society of Clinical Oncology. J Clin Oncol 2002; 20: 2895–903.

Singal PK, Iliskovic N: Doxorubicin-induced cardiomyopathy. N Engl J Med 1998; 339: 900–5.

2 Thromboembolic events

W Jacot, JL Pujol
Hôpital Universitaire Arnaud de Villeneuve, France

Introduction

Thromboembolic disease, also known as venous thromboembolism (VTE), affects approximately 15% of all cancer patients and represents the second leading cause of death in cancer patients.

Etiology

Various factors are associated with an increased risk of thromboembolic disease. There are no clinically reliable coagulation markers able to identify patients who may benefit from prophylaxis but some clinical parameters may indicate the thrombotic risk (Boxes 2.1 and 2.2).

Box 2.1 *Patient/tumor loop*

- Tumor procoagulant activity (tissue factor, cancer procoagulant)
- Inflammatory response (tumor necrosis factor (TNF), interleukin-1 (IL-1))
- Coagulation abnormalities (increased level of fibrinogen and activated coagulation factors, thrombocytosis, platelet activation)

Box 2.2 *Extrinsic factors (endothelial damage, stasis)*

- Cytotoxic agents, thalidomide, hormonal therapy (tamoxifen, acetate medroxyprogesteron), hematopoietic growth factors
- Radiotherapy
- Venous stasis (extrinsic compression), restricted mobility, hospitalization
- Vessel trauma, surgery

Evaluation

Deep venous thrombosis

Clinical evaluation

On the basis of clinical history and physical examination (Table 2.1), ambulatory patients can be classified in one of three probability groups for deep venous thrombosis:

- low-risk group (score < 0, i.e., 5% probability)
- medium-risk group (score 1–3, i.e., 33% probability)
- high-risk group (score > 3, i.e., 85% probability).

Technical evaluation

Cancer patients are considered to belong at least to the medium-risk group.

Plasma D-dimer measurement is only informative in cancer patients. In cases of negativity, it rules out a thromboembolic event. However, no conclusion can be drawn for an elevated plasma D-dimer level.

A diagnosis of deep venous thrombosis may be detected by compression Doppler ultrasonography.

Table 2.1 *Clinical evaluation of deep vein thrombosis*

Clinical feature	Score
Active cancer/anticancer treatment	1
Paralysis, paresis or recent immobilization of the lower extremities	1
Recently bedridden for more than 3 days or major surgery within 4 weeks	1
Localized tenderness along the distribution of the deep venous system	1
Entire leg swollen	1
Calf swelling by more than 3 cm when compared with the asymptomatic leg (measured 10 cm below tibial tuberosity)	1
Pitting edema (greater in the symptomatic leg)	1
Collateral superficial veins (non-varicose)	1
Alternative diagnosis as likely or greater than that of deep venous thrombosis	−2

In patients with symptoms in both legs, the most symptomatic leg is used.

Contrast venography is still considered as the reference test for diagnosis of deep venous thrombosis, but the numerous disadvantages of this technique limit its indication to patients with a negative Doppler ultrasonography with a high suspicion of deep venous thrombosis.

Pulmonary embolism

Clinical evaluation

Individually, clinical examination and simple radiographic and laboratory tests lack sensitivity and specificity. However, the combination of these data allows a more accurate evaluation of the probability of pulmonary embolism (Box 2.3).

Technical examinations

D-dimer measurement is only informative in case of negativity, ruling out a thromboembolic diagnosis. However, no conclusion can be drawn for an elevation of plasma D-dimer level in patients suffering from cancer.

The diagnosis can be made by a positive chest computed tomography (CT) or pulmonary angiogram.

Due to their cancer and/or associated pathologies, the ventilation/perfusion (V/Q) scan must be strictly analyzed in consideration of a high false-positive rate, leading to a lower accuracy in this context. The diagnosis of pulmonary embolism can be excluded by a normal lung perfusion scan.

In case of a diagnosis of pulmonary embolism, an associated deep venous thrombosis might be detected by compression Doppler ultrasonography. Furthermore, an atrial fibrillation (electrocardiogram) in association with hyperthyroidism (thyroid-stimulating hormone) should be excluded.

Pulmonary embolism is classified as massive in case of hypotension or shock; severe hypoxemic respiratory failure; acute right-sided heart dysfunction; or obstruction of the pulmonary vasculature that exceeds 50% as demonstrated by angiogram or V/Q scan. In this setting, a subgroup with the worst prognosis must be individualized: submassive pulmonary embolism, characterized by an echocardiographic acute right-sided heart dysfunction.

Box 2.3 *Checklist for guiding the empirical clinical assessment of probability of pulmonary embolism*

History and risk factors:
- Family or personal history of deep venous thrombosis or pulmonary embolism
- Lower limb venous insufficiency, varicose veins
- Recent trauma or surgery (<1 month)
- Recent immobilization
- Stroke
- Cancer
- Chronic obstructive lung disease
- Heart failure, ischemic heart disease
- Pregnancy or postpartum period
- Estrogen use (contraceptive pill, hormone replacement therapy), tamoxifen, thalidomide

Symptoms:
- Dyspnea
- Chest pain
- Lower limb pain
- Recent dry cough
- Hemoptysis

Physical examination:
- Vital signs (including respiratory rate, heart rate, blood pressure)
- Signs of deep venous thrombosis

Chest X-ray:
- Pleural effusion
- Band atelectasis
- Elevation of hemidiaphragm

Blood gases:
- PaO_2
- $PaCO_2$
- pH
- Alveoloarterial partial oxygen pressure difference

Electrocardiogram:
- S_1Q_3
- Right bundle-branch block
- Other signs of right ventricular strain

Management

Primary prophylaxis

Lower-limb compression

Considering physical methods used to reduce deep venous thrombosis, and more specifically postoperative deep venous thrombosis, there is evidence that external pneumatic compression is an efficient way to reduce deep venous thrombosis, whereas there is no such evidence for elastic stockings.

Low molecular weight heparin

In cancer patients undergoing surgery, low molecular weight heparin is indicated:

- 5000 IU dalteparin or 40 mg enoxaparin subcutaneously started preoperatively and continued once daily postoperatively.

Unfractionated heparin anti-Xa

In cancer patients undergoing surgery, anti-Xa is indicated:

- Unfractioned heparin (UFH) 5000 anti-Xa IU subcutaneously started 2 hours preoperatively and continued for 8–12 hours after surgery.

Coumarin derivatives

In patients treated with chemotherapy:

- Low-dose warfarin, dosed to maintain an INR of 1.3–1.9 has been shown to significantly reduce thromboembolic events in patients with stage IV breast cancer. Further studies are required to confirm these results and to evaluate the benefit of antithrombotic therapies in other tumor types.
- There may be a potential positive influence of anticoagulant treatment on prognosis in various tumor types such as small cell lung cancer. The exact therapeutic impact of anticoagulant therapy as antineoplastic treatment in cancer patients has still to be clearly determined.

Treatment

There is no evidence to treat patients with cancer and thromboembolism differently than patients without cancer.

Deep venous thrombosis

After diagnosis of deep venous thrombosis and in absence of suspicion of pulmonary embolism or clinical severe deep venous thrombosis such as phlegmasia alba dolens, the treatment can be initiated in an outpatient setting. In all other cases, the patient must be hospitalized.

A meta-analysis of treatment trials of venous thromboembolism comparing UFH and low molecular weight heparin in a population of patients with or without cancer showed that low molecular weight heparin therapy results in slightly less recurrent venous thromboembolism, less major bleeding, less thrombus progression and a slightly lower all-cause mortality during the following 3 months.

Low molecular weight heparin should be preferred as first-line therapy. Patients treated at home should be instructed to administer subcutaneous injections and should have a close follow-up. Platelet count must be checked twice weekly during heparin treatment because of heparin-induced thrombocytopenia.

Coumarin therapy should be initiated on day 1. After 4–5 days and when the INR is higher than 2.0 for 2 consecutive days, heparin therapy can be discontinued. Anticoagulation therapy should continue for at least 6 months, although the optimal treatment time is unknown in cancer patients. According to some authors, lifelong treatment must be considered in patients with active cancer disease.

Pulmonary embolism

Heparin

UFH or low molecular weight heparin can be used as first-line therapy for pulmonary embolism. However, there is currently no indication of low molecular weight heparin in massive pulmonary embolism.

UFH should be given by an initial bolus of 5000 IU followed by a 1250 IU/h infusion, with dosage adaptation according to the activated partial thromboplastin time (aPPT) monitoring, with a target aPPT between 2 and 3 × the normal value. In case of heparin resistance, or in case of a spontaneously extended aPPT, it is recommended to adapt UFH dosage to the anti-Xa level, with a target anti-Xa level of 0.4–0.7 IU/ml. Platelet count must be checked twice weekly during heparin treatment.

Oral anticoagulants

Coumarin therapy should be initiated on day 1. After 4–5 days and when the INR is higher than 2.0 for 2 consecutive days, heparin therapy can be discontinued. Anticoagulation therapy should continue for at least 6 months, although the optimal treatment time is unknown. INR must be checked regularly during oral anticoagulant therapy. According to some authors, lifelong treatment must be considered in patients with active cancer disease.

Thrombolysis

Indications

- Massive pulmonary embolism without cardiac arrest.
- Submassive pulmonary embolism (controversial).

Contraindications

Absolute contraindications:

- Active internal bleeding.
- Suspicion of aortic dissection.
- Known traumatic cardiopulmonary resuscitation (CPR).
- Severe hypertension despite medication (>180/110 mmHg).
- Major intracranial events (recent cranial trauma, intracranial neoplasm, known arteriovenous malformation or aneurysm, known or highly suspected intracranial hemorrhage, cerebrovascular accident or transient ischemic accident in the last 6 months).
- Major surgery within the last 14 days.
- Pregnancy.

Relative contraindications:

- Recent trauma or major surgery in the last 2 months.
- Initial but controlled severe hypertension (>180/110 mmHg).
- Peptic ulcer disease.
- Remote history of cerebrovascular accident.
- Known bleeding disorder.
- Renal disease.
- Prolonged CPR.
- Streptokinase in last 6 months (for streptokinase thrombolysis only).

According to some authors, active cancer disease must be considered as a relative contraindication to thrombolytic therapy due to its frequent association

■ Streptokinase	250 000 IU in 20 minutes infusion followed by a 100 000 IU/h 24 hours infusion	
■ Urokinase	4400 IU/kg in 10 minutes infusion followed by a 4400 IU/kg/h 12 hours infusion	
■ rtPA	100 mg in 2-hour infusion	

with bleeding disorders and to the risk of tumor hemorrhage. Food and drug agency (FDA)-approved thrombolysis protocols are given in Box 2.4.

Heparin treatment is initiated after reaching a level of fibrinogen >1 g/L and an aPTT <2 (streptokinase and urokinase), or immediately after the 2-hour infusion of recombinant tissue plasminogen activator (rtPA).

Pulmonary embolectomy (surgical or radiological)

This invasive technique is indicated in massive pulmonary embolism complicated by shock or cardiac arrest.

Recurrent thromboembolism during oral anticoagulation

Guidelines for the anticoagulation strategy in this setting are not standardized. However, in one randomized study, patients with cancer and a recurrent episode of acute, symptomatic proximal deep venous thrombosis, pulmonary embolism or both were treated with low molecular weight heparin (dalteparin) at a dose of 200 IU/kg of body weight subcutaneously once daily for 5–7 days and a coumarin derivative for 6 months (target INR 2.5) or dalteparin alone for 6 months (200 IU/kg once daily for 1 month, followed by a daily dose of approximately 150 IU/kg for 5 months). Dalteparin was more effective than an oral anticoagulant in reducing the risk of recurrent thromboembolism without increasing the risk of bleeding.

If heparin therapy fails, the only option remains the insertion of a vena cava filter.

Complications of antithrombotic therapies

The risk of bleeding during anticoagulation is not statistically different in patients with or without cancer. There is no need to reduce the intensity of anticoagulation in cancer patients in the absence of contraindications.

Hemorrhagic complications due to excessive doses of antithrombotic therapies can be managed as followed:

- UFH and low molecular weight heparin: antagonism by protamine sulfate: 1 mg of protamine sulfate inhibits 100 IU of heparin. Careful determination of the protamine dose must be performed due to the antithrombotic effect of protamine and aPTT should be monitored.
- Oral anticoagulant: antagonism by prothrombin complex concentrate (PCC/PPSB) with INR monitoring.

The platelet count must be monitored twice weekly during UFH and low molecular weight heparin therapy, due to the risk of heparin-induced thrombocytopenia. Delayed heparin-induced thrombocytopenia occurs in approximately 3% of patients receiving intravenous UFH and in 0.5–1% of patients receiving low molecular weight heparin. Heparin treatment must be immediately stopped and another antithrombotic therapy must be initiated.

Conclusion

Venous thromboembolism is a frequent and serious complication of cancer disease and is sometimes caused by anticancer treatment. It is the second leading cause of death in cancer patients and is considered in various tumor types as a bad prognostic factor. Since anticoagulant therapy can lead to treatment delay, cancer patients must be strictly clinically followed in search of venous thromboembolic signs, and prophylaxis must be initiated as soon as complementary risk factors are present. The optimal duration of anticoagulation in patients with active cancer disease and the antineoplastic effect of anticoagulant treatment must be determined by further studies.

Further reading

Dolovich LR, Ginsberg JS, Douketis JD et al: A meta-analysis comparing low-molecular-weight heparins with unfractionated heparin in the treatment of venous thromboembolism: examining some unanswered questions regarding location of treatment, product type, and dosing frequency. Arch Intern Med 2000; 160: 181–8.

Gould MK, Dembitzer AD, Doyle RL et al: Low-molecular-weight heparins compared with unfractionated heparin for treatment of acute deep venous thrombosis. A cost-effectiveness analysis. Ann Intern Med 1999; 130: 789–99.

Lebeau B, Chastang C, Brechot JM et al: Subcutaneous heparin treatment increases survival in small cell lung cancer. "Petites Cellules" Group. Cancer 1994; 74: 38–45.

Lee AY: Cancer and thromboembolic disease: pathogenic mechanisms. Cancer Treat Rev 2002; 28:137–40.

Lee AY, Levine MN: Venous thromboembolism and cancer: risks and outcomes. Circulation 2003; 107(23 Suppl 1):17–21.

Lee AY, Levine MN, Baker RI et al: Low-molecular-weight heparin versus a coumarin for the prevention of recurrent venous thromboembolism in patients with cancer. N Engl J Med 2003; 349: 146–53.

Leizorovicz A: Comparison of the efficacy and safety of low molecular weight heparins and unfractionated heparin in the initial treatment of deep venous thrombosis. An updated meta-analysis. Drugs 1996; 52 (Suppl 7): 30–7.

Letai A, Kuter DJ: Cancer, coagulation, and anticoagulation. Oncologist 1999; 4: 443–9.

Levine M, Hirsh J, Gent M et al: Double-blind randomised trial of a very-low-dose warfarin for prevention of thromboembolism in stage IV breast cancer. Lancet 1994; 343: 886–9.

Ottinger H, Belka C, Kozole G et al: Deep venous thrombosis and pulmonary artery embolism in high-grade non-Hodgkin's lymphoma: incidence, causes and prognostic relevance. Eur J Haematol 1995; 54:186–94.

Perrier A, Miron MJ, Desmarais S et al: Using clinical evaluation and lung scan to rule out suspected pulmonary embolism: Is it a valid option in patients with normal results of lower-limb venous compression ultrasonography? Arch Intern Med 2000; 160: 512–16.

Prandoni P, Piccioli A, Girolami A: Cancer and venous thromboembolism: an overview. Haematologica 1999; 84: 437–45.

Wells PS, Anderson DR, Bormanis J et al: Value of assessment of pretest probability of deep-vein thrombosis in clinical management. Lancet 1997; 350: 1795–8.

3 Superior vena cava syndrome

CN Costovici
Medical Center For Diagnosis and Ambulatory Treatment,
Romania

F Badulescu
University Hospital Craiova, Romania

Introduction

Superior vena cava syndrome (SVCS) is an array of symptoms caused by the obstruction of blood flow through the vena cava superior to the right atrium. The vena cava superior is formed by the union of right and left brachiocephalic veins and empties into the superior-posterior atrium. It is located in the middle of the mediastinum and is in close relationship with structures like the sternum, trachea, right bronchus, aorta, pulmonary artery and the paratracheal and perihilar nodes.

The superior vena cava is thin-walled, compliant and easily compressible vein. When the superior vena cava is fully or partially obstructed, extensive collateral circulation may develop. The most important alternative pathway is the azygos venous system. Other collateral systems are the internal mammary vessels, lateral thoracic veins, paraspinous and esophageal venous network. Subcutaneous veins are also important and their engorgement in the neck and thorax is a typical physical finding.

Etiology

Superior vena cava syndrome may result from compression, invasion or thrombosis of the superior vena cava. Superimposed thrombosis of the superior vena cava may occur secondarily in 30–50% of patients.

In the past, it resulted from inflammatory or benign causes, whereas in more recent series neoplasms account for 80–98%. Lung cancer is the most frequent type, whereas other malignancies include lymphoma, metastatic neoplasm and primary mediastinal tumors (Box 3.1).

Box 3.1 *Principal causes of superior vena cava syndrome*

Lung cancer (52-81%):
- Small cell cancer
- Non-small cell cancer
- Diffuse large cell cancer

Lymphoma (2-20%):
- Lymphoblastic

Metastatic disease to mediastinum (8–10%):
- Breast cancer
- Germ cell cancer
- Gastrointestinal cancers
- Other

Primary mediastinal tumors:
- Thymoma
- Sarcomas (e.g., malignant fibrous hystiocytoma)
- Melanomas
- Thymic carcinoma

Non-malignant causes
- Infectious diseases – syphilis, tuberculosis and histoplasmosis
- Central line thrombus and other iatrogenic causes
- Idiopathic fibrosing mediastinitis
- Congestive heart failure
- Goiter

Evaluation

- The clinical presentation of SVCS may be acute or subacute. A slowly progressive occlusion of the SVC may allow collateral blood flow to develop. An acute obstruction of the blood flow from the head and upper extremities will cause increased venous pressure with symptoms. The severity of SVCS depends on the underlying cause, rapidity of obstruction, concurrent thrombosis, location of obstruction and adequacy of collateral circulation. The most common symptoms and signs of SVCS are summarized in Boxes 3.2 and 3.3. Occult SVCS is uncommon.
- Physical examination may be sufficient to establish the diagnosis of SVCS (see Box 3.3).
- A chest radiograph is usually abnormal. One- to two-thirds of patients have a superior mediastinal mass or widening. In 10–40% of patients, a

Box 3.2 *Symptoms of superior vena cava syndrome*

Dyspnea	Nasal stuffiness
Facial edema	Tongue swelling
Cough	Nausea
Headache	Light headedness
Distorted vision	Stridor
Hoarseness	

Box 3.3 *Signs of superior vena cava syndrome*

Jugular venous distension	Lethargy, stupor and coma
Upper extremity swelling	Syncope
Facial and upper body plethora	Cyanosis
Chemosis	Papilledema
Mental status changes	

right hilar mass is detected. Right-sided pleural effusion is present in approximately 25% of patients. Other common findings include hilar adenopathy and pulmonary masses in 20% of patients. Chest radiograph is normal in 3–15%.

■ Contrast-enhanced CT or MRI is the most cost-effective and accurate imaging study in patients with SVCS to localize the level of SVC obstruction (SVCO), and to show SVC thrombosis, collateral circulation, mediastinal adenopathy or masses.

■ Contrast venography is indicated when surgery is anticipated.

■ Radionuclide venography is comparable to contrast venography in locating the site of obstruction and collateral circulation.

■ Sputum cytology is diagnostic in up to two-thirds of patients with SVCS and small cell lung cancer.

■ Mediastinoscopy and, if necessary, thoracotomy and sternotomy can be justified for diagnosis.

■ A tissue diagnostic is mandatory and is usually obtained via bronchoscopy, fine-needle aspiration, excisional biopsy of a supraclavicular node or CT-directed biopsy of a mass or lymph node in the chest.

Treatment

SVCS is rarely an oncologic emergency and diagnostic work-up should always be performed (Figure 3.1). Only patients with compromised airways, cardiovascular collapse or significantly elevated intracranial pressure are at risk for immediate morbidity and require emergency treatment.

Initial treatment depends upon the diagnosis and symptom progression and includes radiotherapy, chemotherapy, venous bypass, anticoagulation and supportive measures.

Radiotherapy

Radiotherapy is an effective treatment for most malignant causes of SVCS and gives symptomatic relief in 70–90% of patients, with only 10–15% non-responders. In non-small cell lung cancer or neoplasm less sensitive to chemotherapy, treatment with radiotherapy offers effective palliation in 70% of patients.

The fractionation of radiation is important and usually several high-dose fractions (3–4 Gy) are given initially to achieve rapid tumor reduction and symptom relief. High-dose fractions (doses >3 Gy/day) produce an improved response compared with conventional doses of 2 Gy/day.

Chemotherapy

Chemotherapy is indicated in chemosensitive tumors (small cell lung cancer, germ cell tumor, lymphoma) with a rapid regression of signs and symptoms. It is used as single treatment modality or associated with concomitant or subsequent radiotherapy.

Re-evaluation is after 3 courses of chemotherapy and in case of response, the same chemotherapy will be continued for 3 more courses. In case of stable disease or disease progression, an alternative chemotherapy regimen and/or radiotherapy are given.

In non-small cell lung cancer, 60% of patients had relief of SVCS following chemotherapy and/or radiotherapy but 19% of those treated had a recurrence of SVCO.

Anticoagulant or thrombolytic therapy

The use of anticoagulant or thrombolytic therapy is questionable. Because most patients respond to specific therapy, it is not used routinely and remains an option for patients who are not responding or progressing. If a thrombosis

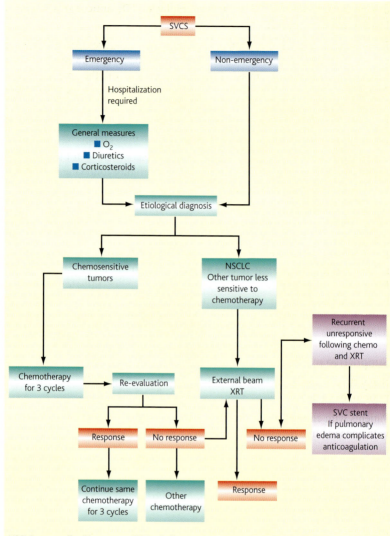

NSCLC: non-small cell lung cancer; XRT: radiotherapy; SVC: superior vena cava

Figure 3.1 Algorithm of treatment in superior vena cava syndrome

can be documented on contrast venography or CT, anticoagulation with heparin may be of benefit.

Fibrinolytic therapy may be effective in patients who developed SVCS on a venous access catheter and is least likely to be beneficial in patients with SVCS due to tumor invasion or compression of the mediastinum. Thrombolysis should be initiated within 7 days after onset of symptoms.

Expandable metal stent

Insertion of a SVC stent may relieve SVCO in 95% patients; 11% of those treated had further SVCO, but recanalization was possible in the majority, resulting in a long-term patency rate of 92%. Morbidity following stent insertion was greater if thrombolytics were administered.

Surgical reconstruction

Surgical reconstruction of the SVC or venous bypass surgery may be useful techniques to palliate symptoms only in selected patients. There has been considerable interest in operative intervention, but results remain controversial. Many techniques such as saphenous-jugular bypass or a prosthetic bypass have been reported. These procedures should be reserved for patients with severe central nervous system symptoms who are not responding to conventional therapy.

Supportive measures

Supportive measures usually allow time to evaluate the pathological specimen prior to initiating specific therapy.

Patients with clinical SVCS often have significant symptomatic improvement with conservative treatment such as elevation of the upper body, oxygen and diuresis (diuretic therapy induces temporary symptomatic improvement but dehydration may result in thrombosis and worsening of the SVCS).

The role of corticosteroids in SVCS is controversial, with limited symptomatic benefit. They are used for a short period and their use is only continued if a response is seen or if there is evidence of cerebral edema.

Stridor or airways obstruction that does not respond to corticosteroids and bronchodilators may require intubation or emergency tracheostomy.

Further reading

Abraham J, Allegra JC: Bethesda Handbook of Clinical Oncology. Baltimore: Lippincott, Williams & Williams, 2001.

Amrah RS, Kennedy MJ: Superior vena cava syndrome. In: Johnston PG, Spence RAJ (eds), Oncologic Emergencies. Oxford: Oxford University Press, 2002: 20–2.

Rowell NP, Gleeson FV: Steroids, radiotherapy, chemotherapy and stents for superior vena caval obstruction in carcinoma of the bronchus: a systematic review. Clin Oncol (R Coll Radiol) 2002; 14: 338–51.

Turnbull ADM: Surgical Emergencies in the Cancer Patient. Chicago: Year Book Medical Publishers, 1987: 303–6.

Yahalom J: Oncologic mergencies, sect.1 SVCS. In: deVita VT, Hellman S, Rosenberg SA (eds), Cancer: Principles and Practice of Oncology, 6th edn. Philadelphia: Lippincott Raven, 2001: pp 2609–15.

Complications of central venous devices

F Andre, E Desruennes
Institut Gustace Roussy, France

Intravascular cathether-related infections

Evaluation

Clinical presentation

- Fever: high sensitivity, poor specificity.
- Inflammation or purulence around the intravascular device.
- Bloodstream infection without other cause.
- Septic shock.
- Sudden onset of symptoms of bloodstream infection soon after initiation of an infusion.
- Others: endocarditis, pulmonary abscess.

A catheter-related infection is clinically suspected in all these clinical situations.

Microbiology

Blood cultures

When a bacteremia secondary to catheter-related infection is suspected, paired blood cultures are drawn through the catheter and a peripheral vein. The diagnosis of catheter-related infection is highly suspected when:

- blood culture from the catheter is positive while the peripheral blood culture is negative
- quantitative difference between the catheter and peripheral blood culture (5- to 10-fold higher colonization of the culture from catheter, or >100 CFU/ml in the culture of blood from catheter)
- there is a differential time of positivity for catheter versus peripheral blood culture (>2 hours).

A catheter-related infection is also suspected when blood culture from a catheter and peripheral blood culture are positive, without any other cause.

When peripheral blood cultures are positive, and blood cultures from the catheter are negative, the probability that the bloodstream infection is related to a catheter infection is low.

Culture of the catheter

- Requires catheter removal.
- A yield of 15 CFU from a catheter by means of semiquantitative culture, or a yield of 10^2 CFU from a catheter by means of quantitative culture, with accompanying signs of local or systemic infection, is indicative of catheter-related infection.

Treatment

Presence of bacteremia

- With complications (septic shock, severe sepsis, thrombophlebitis, septic metastasis) or high risk for complication (heart disease):
  - remove catheter + intravenous antibiotics.
- Without complications, the management is dependent of the pathogen:
  - Coagulase-negative staphylococcus: no removal of catheter + 7–14 days intravenous antibiotics + antibiotic lock for 14 days. In case of persistence of infectious symptoms, complications or deterioration, remove catheter
  - *Staphylococcus aureus*: remove catheter + 14 days intravenous antibiotics (oxacillin or vancomycin) + echocardiography (endocarditis)
  - *Pseudomonas* or multi-resistant Gram-negative bacteria: remove catheter + 14 days intravenous antibiotics
  - Fungal infection: remove catheter + intravenous fluconazole (except for *Candida krusei* or *Candida glabrata*, *Mucor* spp. and *Malassezia furfur*) or amphotericin B.

Local infection without bacteremia

- No abscess, cellulitis, fever or complication: remove catheter + follow-up.
- Local infection + fever: remove catheter + intravenous antibiotics.
- Abscess or cellulitis: empiric intravenous antibiotics + remove catheter.

Special situations

- Septic shock, serious sepsis without shock, neutropenia, thrombophlebitis, endocarditis, abscess in bone, lung, liver or local abscess: empirical intravenous antibiotics (vancomycin + β-lactam ± aminoglycoside in case of septic shock or neutropenia) + remove catheter even without bacterial documentation.

■ Sudden onset of symptoms of bloodstream infection soon after the initiation of infusion:
  – discontinue perfusion
  – peripheral catheter for hydration
  – empirical antibiotics.
  The decision to remove catheter depends on symptoms and pathogen.

Catheter thrombosis

Clinical presentation
■ Edema, fever, arm pain, collateral circulation. In rare cases: superior vena cava syndrome.
■ Check for pulmonary embolism.

Evaluation
Ultrasonography.

Treatment
■ No hospitalization if there is no suspicion of pulmonary embolism or infection and if there is no local complication.
■ Low molecular weight heparin for 5–7 days, followed by:
  – oral anticoagulation therapy
  – continuation of low molecular weight heparin if contraindication for oral anticoagulation therapy or predicted difficulties to equilibrate the international normalized ratio (INR).
■ There is no consensus to remove the catheter: the benefit of catheter removal is unknown.
■ In case of superior vena cava syndrome related to thrombosis, thrombolysis could be discussed with the intensive care unit.
■ Treatment duration:
  – 3 months in case of catheter for adjuvant systemic treatment
  – longer (as long as active cancer disease) in palliative situation.
■ Follow-up: ultrasonography 1 month after starting heparin.

Mechanical complications

Occlusion of central venous access device

Local fibrinolysis: streptokinase 5000 to 10 000 IU in 2 ml saline, applied into the catheter from 30 minutes–12 hours overnight or alteplase: 2 mg in 2 ml saline.

No backward flow

X-ray control:

- if no obvious cause: X-ray + opacification
- if no obvious cause but normal injection without resistance: catheter use is possible
- if fibrin at the catheter tip without thrombosis: local administration of streptokinase or alteplase.

Further reading

Blot F, Nitenberg G, Chachaty E et al: Diagnosis of catheter-related bacteraemia: a prospective comparison of the time to positivity of hub-blood versus peripheral-blood cultures. Lancet 1999; 354: 1071–7.

Mermel LA, Farr BM, Sherertz RJ et al: Infectious Diseases Society of America; American College of Critical Care Medicine; Society for Healthcare Epidemiology of America. Guidelines for the management of intravascular catheter-related infections. Clin Infect Dis 2001; 32: 1249–72.

Timoney JP, Malkin MG, Leone DM: Safe and cost effective use of alteplase for the clearance of occluded central venous access devices. J Clin Oncol 2002; 20: 1918–22.

Verso M, Agnelli G. Venous thromboembolism associated with long-term use of central venous catheters in cancer patients. J Clin Oncol 2003; 21: 3665–75.

Septic shock

E Calvo
Hospital San Jaime, Spain

5

Definition

Sepsis is the systemic inflammatory response to infection and is part of a continuum of injury response, ranging from sepsis to septic shock and multiple organ failure.

Septic shock is diagnosed when there is:

- clinical evidence of infection (fever, chills, hypothermia, leukocytosis, left shift of neutrophils or neutropenia) and
- persistent sepsis-induced hypotension (systolic blood pressure <90 mmHg or a reduction of ≥40 mmHg from baseline), despite volume resuscitation (i.e., vasopressor requirement for sepsis-induced hypotension) and
- evidence of sepsis-related organ hypoperfusion (that may include, but is not limited to lactic acidosis, decreased urine output or altered mental status).

Some cancer patients (elderly patients, patients with uremia or overt immunosuppression) in whom sepsis develops do not become febrile. Early clinical manifestations of sepsis in these patients could consist of subtle changes in mental status, modifications in white cell count or neutrophils percentage or elevated blood glucose levels.

Evaluation and treatment

Septic shock is a life-threatening situation, so priority must be given to the urgent treatment of its cause: the infection. Diagnostic procedures should be performed quickly, without delaying the administration of antibiotics and supportive care to the patient.

Boxes 5.1 and 5.2 summarize the management of these complex patients.

Box 5.1 *Management of the cancer patient with septic shock*

1. **Early stage septic shock**

   Goal: early reversal of the shock, in the first hours.

   Management: early goal-directed therapy.

   1.1 Diagnosis of source of infection and severity of shock.

      - Physical examination, vitals, complete blood analysis.
      - Multiple sampling for cultures and Gram stains.

   1.2 Fluid challenge (colloids or crystalloids, antibiotics, red blood cell transfusions) and oxygen support

      Goals: central venous pressure (CVP) 8–12 mmHg, mean arterial pressure ≥65 mmHg; urine output ≥0.5 ml.kg^{-1}.hr^{-1}; and central venous oxygen saturations ≥70%.

   1.3 Antimicrobial therapy

      Goal: ensure that empiric therapy is effective against the cause of shock.

      - Diagnosis and treatment of the source of infection.
      - Antibiotics administration (a three drug combination against Gram-positive and Gram-negative bacteria and fungi).

   1.4 Intensive insulin therapy

      Goal: glucose levels at <150 mg/dl.

2. **Resistant septic shock**

   Goals: Central venous pressure (CVP) 8–12 mmHg, mean arterial pressure ≥65 mmHg; urine output ≥0.5 ml.kg^{-1}.hr^{-1}; and central venous oxygen saturations ≥70%.

   Management: vasopressor and inotropic agents.

   2.1 Norepinephrine (noradrenaline)

   2.2 Dobutamine

   2.3 Vasopressin

3. **Refractory septic shock**

   3.1 Low-dose corticosteroids

   3.2 Drotrecogin alfa

   3.3 Consider transfer to the Intensive Care Unit

Box 5.2 *Additional support for the stabilized patient*

- Enteral nutrition (if not contraindicated)
- Deep venous thrombosis prophylaxis (if not contraindicated)
- Stress ulcer prophylaxis
- Granulocyte colony-stimulating factor, if neutropenic patient
- Adjust antibiotic regimen according to microbiology results

Antimicrobial therapy

Early initiation of appropriate antibiotics and adequate control of the source of the infection are key components of septic shock treatment. Basic principles are to ensure that empiric therapy is effective against the pathogen and it is initiated as quickly as possible, and that the optimum target levels of antibiotics are achieved rapidly.

Diagnosis of infection

- Meticulous physical assessment of common sites of infection (mouth, pharynx, respiratory tract, skin and soft tissue, perineal area, urinary and gastrointestinal tract, and exit sites of peripheral or venous catheters) should be done immediately.
- A complete blood analysis profile (complete blood count, biochemistry, coagulation times, electrolytes, arterial gases) should be done immediately.
- Samples for cultures and stains for bacteria and fungi (from urine, stool, drainage sites, sputum, blood (if a central venous catheter is in place, collect the cultures from each lumen as well as from a peripheral vein), and cerebrospinal fluid if suspicion of a central nervous system (CNS) infection) should be taken as soon as possible. Cultures, especially from blood, should be done ideally after onset of fever or chills and before the first dose of antibiotics.
- When a central venous catheter is suspected as the source of septic shock, the catheter should be removed, replaced at a distant site and sent for culture.
- Investigation of suspected pneumonia should include a chest radiography (if negative, an early computed tomography) and pleural effusion aspiration and evaluation.

- If intra-abdominal sepsis is suspected an initial ultrasound or a computed tomography should be performed urgently. Collections identified should be drained under radiological control and samples sent for Gram-staining and culture.

Antibiotics in septic shock

- There is an important lack of studies of empirical antibiotic therapy in critically ill cancer patients with septic shock. It is fundamental that empirical antibiotic therapy is effective against most of the theoretical potential pathogens.
- The number of infections in cancer patients caused by Gram-positive bacteria and fungi has increased markedly in the last 15 years, while the number of infections caused by Gram-negative bacteria has remained constant. Based on these assumptions, as well as on the general rules for the treatment of infections in the cancer patient, an initial wide-spectrum three-drug therapy regimen is recommended, including two antibacterial agents (Gram-positive and Gram-negative bacteria) and one antifungal drug.
- Different regimens of intravenous antibiotics can be considered, depending on the experience of the oncologist and the availability of drugs:
    - a third- or fourth-generation cephalosporin (ceftazidime or cefepime) or a carbapenem (imipenem-cilastin or meropenem), plus
    - a glycopeptide (vancomycin or teicoplanin in case of renal impairment), plus
    - amphotericin B (in case of renal impairment, administer liposomal amphotericin B).
- Additional coverage for patients at specific pathogens risks:
    - Patients with suspected pneumonia by *Pneumocystis carinii* should receive trimethoprim-sulfamethoxazole.
    - Anaerobic coverage (metronidazole, clindamycin, chloramphenicol) should be considered in patients with abdominal abscesses or acute abdominal pain suggestive of typhlitis.
    - Aminoglycoside administration (i.e., tobramycin, or amikacin) for the neutropenic patient, and also if a *Pseudomonas aeruginosa* or Gram-negative sepsis is suspected.
    - If interstitial pneumonia is observed in a transplanted patient or in a patient being chronically treated with corticosteroids, ganciclovir is also added.
- Once the results of the cultures are known, the antibiotic regimen has to be adjusted according to the antibiogram.

Hemodynamic support

Early aggressive therapy to optimize cardiac function, blood pressure and oxygen delivery (central venous pressure of 8–12 mmHg, mean arterial pressure of more than 65 mmHg, and central venous oxygen saturations of more than 70%), including infusions of colloid or crystalloid, vasoactive and/or inotropic agents and transfusions of red blood cells to increase oxygen delivery during the first 6 "golden hours" of septic shock are associated with an absolute decrease of 15% in mortality rate compared with less aggressive standard resuscitation therapy.

Fluid resuscitation

- Fluid challenge should be titrated to the clinical endpoints of blood pressure (arbitrary values of a systolic blood pressure of 90 mmHg or a mean arterial blood pressure of 60–65 mmHg).
  Central venous pressure is initially required to evaluate the relationship between intravascular volume and cardiac function, targeting absolute values between 12 mmHg. In the absence of central hemodynamic monitoring, bolus fluid therapy (250–1000 ml over 5–15 minutes (min)) should be repeated as long as the patient remains hypotensive or until early clinical manifestation of pulmonary edema occurs (crackles on lung auscultation or a drop in oxyhemoglobin saturation).
- Although more expensive, colloids are possibly preferred with respect to crystalloids if hypotension is immediately life-threatening, since less fluid is required to achieve resuscitation goals, offering a more rapid correction of volume deficit with less edema.
- Red blood cell transfusion, as needed to maintain hemoglobin levels between 7.0 and 9.0 g/dl in patients with septic shock, are recommended, since this degree of anemia is usually well tolerated in most patients and allows a correct oxygen delivery.

Vasopressor and inotropic agents

- When fluid challenge fails to restore an adequate arterial pressure and organ perfusion, therapy with vasopressor agents should be started to reach these goals. Vasopressors are also required transiently to sustain life and maintain perfusion in the face of life-threatening hypotension even when cardiac filling pressures are not elevated.
- A combination of inotrope and vasopressor agents is usually chosen. Albeit there are different valid drugs and regimens, the combination of

norepinephrine (noradrenaline) and dobutamine appears to be more predictable and appropriate to the goals of septic shock therapy.

- Norepinephrine is a more potent agent than dopamine in refractory septic shock. Its potential advantages compared with dopamine include minimal tachycardia response and no interference with the hypothalamic–pituitary axis. Norepinephrine markedly improves mean arterial pressure and glomerular filtration. This is particularly true in the high output and low resistance state of many septic shock patients. Its recommended dose ranges from 1 μg/kg/min to 30 μg/kg/min.

- Dobutamine increases cardiac index combined with increases in stroke volume and heart rate. In the presence of severe depression of cardiac contractility and decreased cardiac output despite fluid resuscitation and vasopressor therapy, dobutamine may be considered, at doses ranging from 2 μg/kg/min to 28 μg/kg/min.

- Septic shock-associated exhaustion of neurohypophyseal stores due to intense and prolonged stress stimulation may lead to a relative vasopressin deficiency along with enhanced sensitivity. In patients requiring high-dose vasopressors, especially when blood pressure remains inadequate, vasopressin 0.01–0.04 units/min could be given.

Airway and oxygen support

- Provide adequate supplemental oxygen to maintain an O_2 saturation of 90% through use of simple oxygen delivery systems (i.e., nasal cannula or face mask). In patients with sepsis-related acute respiratory distress syndrome, avoid the use of noninvasive positive-pressure ventilation.

- When indicated, transfer the patient early to the Intensive Care Unit for placement of an endotracheal tube and mechanical ventilation. Indications include severe dyspnea (respiratory rate >40 bpm, use of accessory muscles), altered mental status and severe hypoxemia despite supplemental oxygen.

Immunological therapy

- Corticosteroids are recommended during "refractory" septic shock at low doses (200–300 mg of intravenous hydrocortisone every 6 hours or by continuous infusion every day) plus 50 μg of fludrocortisone orally, for 7 days or more (up to 10 days) and then with subsequent tapering of the dose according to hemodynamic status. This has been shown to decrease absolute mortality in 10% and vasopressor use, especially in those patients with evidence of relative adrenal insufficiency (i.e., a bad response to ACTH stimulation test), who are usually those requiring high-dose or increasing vasopressor therapy within the first 6 hours of septic shock.

- Inflammatory reactions and overt clinical or subclinical manifestations of disseminated intravascular coagulation are present in essentially all patients with septic shock. Drotrecogin alfa (recombinant activated protein C) has an anticoagulant and profibrinolytic effect, as well as an anti-inflammatory effect and produces a significant absolute reduction of 13% in mortality in septic shock patients. It is given in a dose of 24 µg/kg/hour and is recommended in patients with the most severe organ compromise and the highest likelihood of death with an INR <3 and platelet count >30000/mm^3. It major side effect is an increased risk for severe hemorrhages.

- Granulocyte colony-stimulating factors have been shown to shorten the duration of neutropenia, and their use is indicated in the setting of septic shock in neutropenic patients (5 mg/kg subcutaneously, daily, until neutrophil recovery).

Other supportive therapies

Insulin therapy

- It has been demonstrated that intensive insulin therapy that maintained the blood glucose level at 80–110 mg/dl resulted in lower morbidity and mortality (15% absolute reduction) among critically ill patients with sepsis than did conventional therapy that maintained the blood glucose level at 180–200 mg/dl.

- Therefore, it is reasonable to control blood glucose more tightly in critically ill patients. A continuous infusion of insulin (to a maximal dose arbitrarily set at 50 IU of Actrapid HM/hour), with the use of a pump, should be started if the blood glucose level exceeds 110 mg/dl, and the infusion is to be adjusted to maintain normoglycemia or, at least, glucose levels below 150 mg/dl. Be aware of hypoglycemic brain injury in attempting to maintain the blood glucose level within normal limits.

Deep venous thrombosis (DVT) prophylaxis

Stabilized septic shock patients who do not have a contraindication to heparin use (i.e., thrombocytopenia, severe coagulopathy, active bleeding, recent intracerebral hemorrhage, administration of drotrecogin alfa or other anticoagulants) should receive DVT prophylaxis, considering the presence of independent risk factors for DVT in these patients, preferably with low molecular weight heparin at recommended doses (i.e., enoxaparin 40 mg subcutaneously once daily).

Nutritional support

Early and complete enteral nutrition is the preferred method of nutritional support for the critically ill patient, once the patient's condition is stable.

Stress ulcer prophylaxis

Septic patients have multiple risk factors of stress ulcer bleeding. Several trials have confirmed the efficacy of antacids, sucralfate, histamine-2 receptor antagonists or proton-pump inhibitors.

Platelet support

Administer platelets when counts are $<5000/mm^3$ regardless of bleeding. Transfuse platelets when counts are 5000 to $30\,000/mm^3$ and there is significant bleeding risk. Platelet counts of more than $50\,000/mm^3$ are required for surgery or invasive procedures.

Further reading

Dellinger RP: Cardiovascular management of septic shock. Crit Care Med 2003; 31: 946–55.

Dellinger RP, Carlet JM, Masur H et al: Surviving sepsis campaign: guidelines for management of severe sepsis and septic shock. Intensive Care Med 2004; 30: 536–55.

Hotchkiss RS, Karl IE: The pathophysiology and treatment of sepsis. N Engl J Med 2003; 348: 138–50.

International Sepsis Forum: Guidelines for the management of severe sepsis and septic shock. Intensive Care Med 2001; 27 (Suppl 1): 134.

Sharma S, Kumar A: Septic shock, multiple organ failure, and acute respiratory distress syndrome. Curr Opin Pulm Med 2003; 9: 199–209.

Varanasi NL, MacArthur RD: Infections: etiology, treatment, and prevention. In: Skeel RT (ed.), Handbook of Cancer Chemotherapy. Philadelphia: Lippincott, Williams and Wilkins, 2003: 581–602.

Extravasation of chemotherapy

F Andre
Institut Gustave Roussy, France

D Schrijvers
ZNA Middelheim, Belgium

Introduction

Extravasation is defined either as the escape of a chemotherapeutic agent from a vessel into the surrounding tissues by leakage or as an involuntary injection of a drug into the tissues. The frequency of extravasation in adults is considered to be between 0.1% and 6%. The severity of tissue injury is dependent on the type and concentration of the chemotherapeutic agent and the quantity injected.

Cytotoxic agents may be classified as irritants or vesicants (Box 6.1).

Box 6.1 *Vesicants and irritants*

Vesicant drugs
- ■ Alkylating agents: mechlorethamine
- ■ Anthracyclines: Daunorubicin, doxorubicin, epirubicin, idarubicin
- ■ Others: dactinomycin, mitomycin C
- ■ Vinca alkaloids: vinblastine, vincristine, vinorelbine
- ■ Taxanes: docetaxel, paclitaxel

Irritant drugs
- ■ Alkylating agents: carmustine, dacarbazine, carboplatin, cisplatin, cyclophosphamide, ifosfamide, melphalan, oxaliplatin, thiothepa
- ■ Antimetabolites: cytarabine, fludarabine, 5-fluorouracil, gemcitabine, methotrexate, raltitrexed
- ■ Others: bleomycin, etoposide, irinotecan

Symptoms

Irritants are drugs that can cause an inflammatory reaction, aching, swelling, pain or phlebitis at the injection site or along the vein. They may cause sclerosis and hyperpigmentation along the vein, burning, local warmth, discomfort, erythema or tenderness. These symptoms are self-limiting and there are no long-term sequelae.

Vesicants are drugs that may cause severe and lasting tissue injury and necrosis. Symptoms may arise immediately after extravasation or appear after several days or weeks. Patients may complain of pain or local burning at the infusion site, mild erythema, itching or swelling. Over time, the symptoms of erythema and pain may increase and a discoloration and induration of the skin, dry desquamation or blistering may develop. In case of a significant extravasation, necrosis, eschar formation and ulceration with involvement of underlying tissues may occur. The indolent ulceration lacks granulation tissue formation and there is little peripheral re-epithelialization.

Prevention

The most important approach to extravasation is prevention. Prevention of extravasation takes into account several factors.

- Written guidelines for handling cytotoxic agents and procedures in case of extravasation should be present in all departments where chemotherapy is administered.
- An extravasation kit, with all the necessary material and drugs to treat an extravasation, should be present.
- There should be a form to report an extravasation to the authorities (hospital direction, legal department, nursing department).
- Persons responsible for administering cytotoxic drugs should be informed and educated about the drugs and the problems they may cause in case of extravasation and the procedures to follow.
- A cytotoxic agent should not be administered in an extremity if within the previous 48 hours there was a venopuncture above the place of insertion of the catheter.
- For vesicant drugs, the placement of a subcutaneous device before starting chemotherapy is advisable; in case of infusions of longer duration (e.g. more than 1-hour infusions), the placement of a subcutaneous device is obligatory.

- Drugs should never be administered by a butterfly needle and even in case of a bolus injection or a short infusion, a catheter has to be inserted into a vein.
- Small and fragile veins should be avoided.
- The catheter should never be inserted in a limb that is affected by lymphedema or has a neurologic weakness. Veins adjacent to tendons, nerves or arteries should be avoided, while areas of high venous pressure should not be used.
- If the drugs are given by slow bolus injection by peripheral infusion, the placement of the catheter should be in the forearm and not on the hand. In case of extravasation, the tissues and muscles in the forearm may prevent involvement of ligaments, nerves and bone.
- Before administering a cytotoxic agent, the catheter is flushed by a free-flowing infusion with sodium chloride 0.9% or glucose 5% solution for at least 5 minutes. At the end of the administration of a cytotoxic drug, the same procedure is repeated.
- The patient is informed that, in case of pain or other discomfort, the nurse should be informed immediately.
- The exact position of the catheter is checked by aspiration of blood. The drug is then slowly injected.
- In case of complaints by the patient, the administration is stopped, the nurse aspirates as much as possible of the injected drug, stops the infusion, leaves the catheter in place and calls for a physician.
- The physician gives instructions on how to deal with the event and may start a treatment for extravasation.
- The event and the treatment procedure should be noted in the patient's file and on the extravasation form.

Treatment of extravasation

General principles

The type of treatment for extravasation is dependent on the drug.

Extravasation of an irritant

- The catheter may be removed.
- The affected extremity is elevated.
- Cold or warm compresses may be applied. Hot packs are believed to cause vasodilatation, leading to the dilution of the extravasated drug. Cold packs may cause venous constriction, leading to localization of the drug and

therefore increased degradation of toxic metabolites. They may also reduce local inflammation and pain.

- Inflammation may be treated with local anti-inflammatory drugs (corticosteroids).
- Pain should be treated by analgesics.

Extravasation of a vesicant

- Chemotherapy infusion is stopped.
- The catheter is left in place.
- An antidote may be injected, depending on the extravasated drug.
- The affected extremity is kept elevated and a cold or hot pack is applied. In case of extravasation with vinca alkaloids, a hot pack is applied. For all other vesicants, cold packs are indicated.

Ulceration or continued swelling, erythema and pain

A surgical treatment must be discussed with the surgeon.

Specific treatment according to the drug

Prevention of damage

Anthracyclines

- Dimethyl sulfoxide (DMSO): two prospective studies have suggested that the topical application of DMSO may be effective in this situation. In a prospective study, 17 patients were treated with topical DMSO. It was applied immediately after extravasation, covering twice the area affected by the extravasation. This treatment was repeated twice daily for 14 days. No ulceration developed and no surgical intervention was necessary.

  In another prospective study, 69 patients suffering from an anthracycline extravasation, 99% DMSO was applied topically every 8 hours for 7 days in combination with intermittent cooling (1 hour 3 times daily). This treatment proved to be safe and effective, with ulceration developing in only one patient. Side effects were mild local burning and a characteristic breath odor due to DMSO.

- Dexrazoxane has been advocated for the treatment of anthracycline extravasation. It is given intravenously (dexrazoxane 1000 mg/m^2 within 5 hours of extravasation on day 1; 1000 mg/m^2 on day 2; 500 mg/m^2 on day 3) within 3–6 hours after anthracycline extravasation.

- Flushing of the region after placement of a subcutaneous canula with saline may be of benefit.

Taxanes

Both docetaxel and paclitaxel have been reported to cause tissue damage after extravasation. Several reports indicate that docetaxel may cause erythema, blistering and pain. Conservative management resulted in complete recovery after 4 weeks, whereas the dilution with subcutaneous saline, local hypothermia and topical DMSO (3 times every 45 minutes), corticosteroids or diclofenac were effective in restricting inflammation.

In an animal model, paclitaxel proved to cause skin ulceration and necrosis, proving its vesicant character. A treatment with intradermal hyaluronidase (15 units) diluted in saline was effective in preventing paclitaxel-induced ulceration. Topical treatment as topical DMSO, cooling or heating had no beneficial effect.

Mitomycin C

Mitomycin C is a vesicant that may cause distant and delayed ulcerations. Toxicity of mitomycin C can be prevented by topical application of DMSO.

Vinca alkaloids

Vinblastine, vincristine and vinorelbine cause tissue damage after extravasation:

- apply hot packs
- use dilution with saline or hyaluronidase (150–1500 units subcutaneously in surrounding tissues).

Nitrogen mustard or mechlorethamine

Immediate subcutaneous administration of 2 ml of a 0.17 molar sodium thiosulfate solution (4 ml of 10% sodium thiosulfate USP and 6 ml sterile water for injection).

Treatment of ulcerations

Granulocyte (macrophage) colony-stimulating factor (GM-CSF)

One patient has been reported who developed two doxorubicin-induced ulcerations. One ulcer was treated with weekly GM-CSF at a dose of 400 µg subcutaneously for 3 weeks and did heal by the 4th week. The second ulcer was treated with GM-CSF, but no improvement was seen.

Surgical approach

- Early surgical resection with delayed closure of the wound within 24 hours to 1 week after extravasation is indicated in patients with severe pain. The extent of surgery may be determined by fluorescence microscopy. Excision of all fluorescence-positive tissues led to less late sequels when performed within 7 hours. The wound may be temporarily covered with a biologic dressing. Once the wound is clean, a delayed application of a skin graft (split-thickness) may be applied after 2–3 days.

- A conservative approach is an option since only one-third of vesicants will give rise to an ulceration. Continued swelling, erythema and pain without ulceration, persisting after conservative therapy or the presence of large areas of tissue necrosis or skin ulcerations are indications for surgery. In this case, surgery is usually performed 2–3 weeks after extravasation.

Conclusion

Extravasation is a severe complication of chemotherapy. Prevention by adequate guidelines of chemotherapy administration and training of nurses is of importance. In case of extravasation, the correct treatment according to the specific drug should be given (Table 6.1).

Table 6.1 Guidelines for antidote use after extravasation

Drug	Antidote	Advice
Anthracyclines	DMSO	Apply locally as soon as possible and repeat every 8 h for 7 days
	Dexrazoxane	1000 mg/m^2 i.v. within 5 h of extravasation on day 1, 1000 mg/m^2, day 2, 500 mg/m^2 on day 3
		Ice packs
Mechlorethamine	Sodium thiosulfate	2 ml of a solution of 4 ml sodium thiosulfate + 6 ml sterile water for injection s.c.
Vinca alkaloids	Hyaluronidase	150–1500 U s.c.
		Hot packs

DMSO, dimethyl sulfoxide; i.v., intravenously; s.c., subcutaneously.

Further reading

Albanell J, Baselga JL: Systemic therapy emergencies. Semin Oncol 2000; 27: 347–61.

Alley E, Green R, Schuchter L: Cutaneous toxicities of cancer therapy. Curr Opin Oncol 2002; 14: 212–16.

Ener RA, Meglathery SB, Styler M: Extravasation of systemic hemato-oncological therapies. Ann Oncol 2004; 15: 858–62.

Fenchel K, Karthaus M: Cytotoxic drug extravasation. Antibiot Chemother 2000; 50: 144–8.

Schrijvers DL: Extravasation: a dreaded complication of chemotherapy. Ann Oncol 2003; 14(Suppl 3): 26–30.

7 Spinal cord compression

G A López
Hospital San Carlos, Argentina

Introduction

Spinal cord compression (SCC) is one of the most devasting complications in cancer patients, occurring when a primary or metastatic tumor produces a mass effect on the spinal cord with neurologic deficit. Spinal metastases frequently grow in the posterior part of the vertebral bodies and compress the anterior structures of the cord. Tumors can also arise from the posterior arch, affecting the posterior aspect of the spinal cord. Moreover, paravertebral tumors may invade first the intervertebral foramina and then the spinal canal, producing a posterolateral compression of the spinal cord.

Etiology

Most patients already have a confirmed diagnosis of malignancy, but in others SCC can be the initial manifestation of cancer. Differential diagnoses to be considered, based on the clinical history and technical evaluation, are vertebral tuberculosis, osteomyelitis, epidural hematomas, herniated intervertebral disks and spondylosis.

The most frequently involved site is the thoracic spine, followed by the lumbar and the cervical spine, although multiple metastases are usually found. Among the tumor types most often observed to compromise the spine are breast, lung, prostate and renal cancer, multiple myeloma and sarcoma.

Expanding tumors can produce direct mechanical damage to the spinal cord and may also produce vertebral fracture, with bone fragments displacement into the spinal canal compressing the cord. In addition, an ischemic mechanism of injury also exists that involves venous plexus obstruction and vasogenic edema by production of vascular endothelial growth factor (VEGF) and prostaglandin E_2 (PGE_2). Subsequent compression of the small arterioles and capillary network causes more ischemia to the white matter, leading to infarction and permanent neurologic damage.

BMA Library

BMA House, Tavistock Square, London WC1H 9JP

British Medical Association
BMA House
Tavistock Square
London
WC1H 9JP

CERTIFICATE OF POSTAGE RECEIPT to be obtained and retained. You are liable for any lost items.

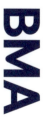

BMA

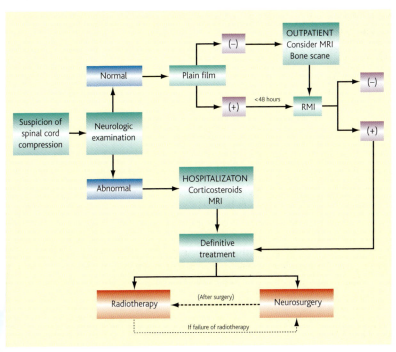

Figure 7.1 Spinal cord compression flowchart

Evaluation of spinal cord compression

Spinal cord compression must always be considered, since early decompressive measures are crucial to preserve neurologic function and quality of life. Less than 15% of patients with a late diagnosis will recover neurologically.

■ Back pain is usually the first symptom that precedes diagnosis. It can be local, radicular or both, depending on the location of the tumor. Pain is usually worsened by straining, coughing, movement and recumbency. Sometimes it is possible to detect the level of the affected site by gentle spine percussion.
Sensory dysfuction, weakness, loss of sphincter control and finally paralysis are the subsequent events that often progress rapidly.

■ Physical examination must include flexor and extensor motor assessment, delimitation of the sensory level and evaluation of the sphincter tone.

- Plain radiography is simple and useful for a first quick evaluation and gives important information, about the affected vertebra such as erosion or collapse.
- Magnetic resonance imaging (MRI) is the imaging technique of choice and is used to detect the location and extension of the compressing tumor. When gadolinium-enhanced MRI is used, paraspinous masses and intramedullary tumors can also be detected.
  Whenever possible, it is preferable to study the entire spine with MRI, since more than one vertebra can be affected by metastases.
- Myelography and computed tomography (CT) are used to evaluate patients with SCC when MRI is not available or contraindicated. They are less sensitive and have less specificity compared with MRI.
  Although myelography by lumbar puncture can detect the level of cord compression, a CT scan delineates the affected spine. Myelography is an invasive method and is less helpful to detect intramedullary and paravertebral tumors. Besides, more punctures must be performed when there is a complete blockade to evaluate the rest of the canal.
- A biopsy guided by CT or MRI can be carried out when histological diagnosis is needed, in the absence of neurologic dysfunction.

Patients with back pain, but without neurologic findings and normal plain films of the spine, can be further evaluated with MRI and bone scan as outpatients.

Patients with normal neurologic examination, but with plain films showing erosion, loss of pedicles or collapse, should be evaluated without delay, preferably with MRI.

Treatment

Patients with neurological symptoms

- Immediate hospitalization.
- Pain control with analgesics.
- Intravenous administration of dexamethasone, 8–10 mg every 6 hours, while emergent evaluation and decompressive measures start (corticosteroids reduce edema and frequently improve the neurologic status). After 48–72 hours, the dose can be reduced to 4–8 mg orally every 6 hours, tapering the dose after 4 days. If neurologic functions deteriorate after reducing corticosteroids, the dose should be restored to a prior effective level.

- Indications for surgery:
  - Spinal compression by bone fragments.
  - Unknown etiology of spinal cord compression and tissue sample is needed in patients with rapid neurological deterioration.
  - Tumor is not responding to radiotherapy.
- Type of surgery:
  - Posterior compression of spinal cord: simple laminectomy.
  - Compression due to vertebral body: anterior decompression, methylmethacrylate replacement and mechanical stabilization since simple laminectomy may lead to spinal instability. Patients should have a good performance status for this procedure.
- Radiotherapy after surgery, if there is not contraindication.

Patients with back pain or with a normal neurologic examination but abnormal radiology

- Pain control with analgesics.
- Corticosteroids can be avoided in patients with no neurologic findings.
- Radiotherapy is the recommended treatment for the majority of patients with SCC, specially for those with slow evolution of symptoms, compromise of cauda equina or widely metastatic disease. It is given in fractions of 25–30 cGy to a total dose of 3000–3500 cGy. Prior radiation treatment on the site excludes from new radiotherapy.
- Hormonal treatment and chemotherapy may also be considered for adults with sensitive tumors and widespread disease, usually after radiotherapy or surgery.
- In children, chemotherapy is frequently the initial treatment with chemosensitive tumors (Ewing's sarcoma, Wilms' tumor or neuroblastoma), in order to avoid the deleterious effects from radiotherapy on spine development. Laminectomy is accepted in this population when emergent decompression is needed.

Complications

Due to the morbidity of spinal cord compression, the lifestyle of patients can worsen dramatically, specially if paraplegia develops. Prognosis depends on the underlying malignancy and complications due to immobilization and other medical problems.

Further reading

Bell GR: Surgical treatment of spinal tumors. Clin Orthop 1997; 335: 54.

Bilsky MH, Lis E, Raizer J, Lee H, Boland P: The diagnosis and treatment of metastatic spinal tumors. Oncologist 1999; 4: 459.

Black P: Spinal epidural tumors. In: Wilkins RH, Rengachary SS (eds), Neurosurgery. New York: McGraw-Hill, 1985: 1062.

Boogerd W, Van der Sande JJ: Treatment of complications: diagnosis and treatment of spinal cord compression in malignant disease. Cancer Treat Rep 1993; 19; 129.

Gilbert RW, Kim J-H, Posner JB: Epidural spinal cord compression from metastatic tumor: diagnosis and treatment. Ann Neurol 1978; 3: 40.

Helweg-Larsen S: Clinical outcome in metastatic spinal cord compression. A prospective study of 153 patients. Acta Neurol Scand 1996; 94: 269.

Helweg-Larsen S, Sorensen PS: Symptoms and signs in metastatic spinal compression: a study of progression from first symptom until diagnosis in 153 patients. Eur J Cancer 1994; 30A: 396.

Husband DJ: Malignant spinal cord compression: prospective study of delays in referral and treatment. BMJ 1998; 317: 18.

Kato A, Ushio Y, Hayakawa T et al: Circulatory disturbance of the spinal cord with epidural neoplasm in rats. J Neurosurg 1985; 63: 260.

Leviov M, Dale J, Stein M et al: The management of metastatic spinal cord compression: a radiotherapeutic success ceiling. Int J Radiat Oncol Biol Phys 1993; 27: 31.

Li KC, Poon PY: Sensitivity and specificity of MRI in detecting malignant spinal cord compression and in distinguishing malignant from benign compression fractures of vertebrae. Magn Reson Imaging 1988; 6: 547.

Loblaw DA, Laperriere NJ: Emergency treatment of malignant extradural spinal cord compression: an evidence-based guideline. J Clin Oncol 1998; 16: 1613.

Maranzano E, Latini P, Beneventi S et al: Radiotherapy without steroids in selected metastatic spinal cord compression patients. A phase II trial. Am J Clin Oncol 1996; 19: 179.

Solberg A, Bremnes RM: Metastatic spinal cord compression: diagnostic delay, treatment, and outcome. Anticancer Res 1999; 19: 677.

Complications of brain metastases

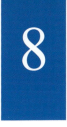

F Cappuzzo
Bellaria Hospital, Italy

Introduction

Brain metastases are estimated to occur in 10–30% of cancer patients and two-thirds of them become symptomatic during their lifetime. Although every solid tumor may spread to the brain, the risk of developing brain metastases is higher in lung cancer, breast cancer and malignant melanoma patients (Table 8.1). Breast cancer patients develop brain metastases in about 10–20% of cases, while brain involvement occurs in about 20–40% of cases of non-small cell lung cancer and 12–20% of cases in melanoma.

At diagnosis, about 10% of patients with small cell lung cancer present with brain metastases, which rises to 20% during therapy and to 50% at autopsy. Several findings suggest that the incidence of brain metastases is rising, as a result of advances in imaging procedures and improvements in therapy, which leaves more cancer patients at risk as survival increases.

Table 8.1 *Incidence of brain metastases in cancer patients (%)*

Primary tumor	Primary tumor incidence	Brain metastases incidence
Breast	181.000	28.600
Lung	168.000	44.200
Colon	156.000	7.000
Prostate	132.000	7.000
Malignant lymphomas	44.400	1.800
Melanoma	32.000	11.800
Pancreas	28.300	1.100

Evaluation and diagnosis

Brain metastases may cause signs and symptoms due to their localization or to the increased intracranial pressure. Presence of brain metastases should be suspected in all cancer patients who develop neurologic symptoms. Progressive neurologic dysfunction is usually related to a gradually expanding tumor mass and associated edema or to the development of obstructive hydrocephalus (Table 8.2).

- Patients may complain of headache, cognitive disturbances, altered mental status and focal weakness. Patients suffer from nausea and vomiting. In 7% of patients with brain metastases there are no symptoms.
- Clinical examination may show focal neurologic signs as aphasia, hemiplegia, hemisensory loss, visual abnormalities and seizures. Other signs are stiff neck, papilledema, pupillary and eye movement abnormalities, hypertension and bradycardia. Patients may lose consciousness.
- Diagnosis is made by computed tomography (CT) scan or magnetic resonance (MRI). Clinical evidence and controlled clinical trials indicate that MRI is more sensitive than CT scan and facilitates early detection of brain metastases.

Analysis of prognostic factors from three Radiation Therapy Oncology Group (RTOG) brain metastases trials identified 3 prognostic classes (Table 8.3). Median survival for class 1 patients was 7.1 months and only 4.2 and 2.3 months for class 2 and 3 patients, respectively. Patients with brain tumors from breast cancer have a longer median survival time than do patients who have brain metastases from other primary tumors such as lung, melanoma or colorectal.

Table 8.2 Symptoms of brain metastases

Symptom prevalence	Incidence (%)
Headache	35–50
Nausea/vomiting	30–40
Asthenia	35–40
Seizure	15–20
Dizziness	10–20
Ataxia	15–20
Aphasia	15–20

Table 8.3 *RTOG Prognostic criteria*

Class	Karnofsky performance status (%)	Age < 65 years, controlled primary tumor, no extracranial disease
1	≥70	Yes
2	≥70	No
3	<70	Yes or no

Treatment

■ Whole brain radiotherapy associated with supportive care remains the standard treatment for all patients with multiple symptomatic brain metastases or with isolated symptomatic brain metastasis in the presence of uncontrolled extracranial disease.

■ Chemotherapy represents the optimal starting therapy in chemosensitive patients with asymptomatic multiple or isolated brain metastases with disseminated disease (Box 8.1).

■ Surgery followed by whole brain radiotherapy may be indicated in patients with controlled extracranial disease, a good performance status and an isolated brain metastasis.

For a long time, supportive care (high-dose corticosteroids and anticonvulsant drugs) and whole brain radiotherapy have been identified as standard treatment for patients with brain metastases. In fact, low life expectancy and the presence of the blood–brain barrier have been considered as contraindications for more aggressive therapies such as chemotherapy.

More recent reports indicate that several drugs such as platinum derivatives, etoposide, teniposide, gemcitabine, irinotecan and topotecan pass the blood–brain barrier and are active against brain metastases (Table 8.4). Several phase II trials that evaluated the activity of different chemotherapy regimens in

Box 8.1 *Active drugs for brain metastases*

Cisplatin	Ifosfamide
Carboplatin	Fotemustine
Etoposide	Temozolomide
Teniposide	

Table 8.4 Main studies evaluating the role of chemotherapy for brain metastases

Reference	Number	Primary tumor	Chemotherapy	Response rate (%)
Rosner	100	Breast	EDX/5FU/Pred ± MTX/VCR	50
Rosner	26	Breast	EDX/5FU/Pred EDX/5FU/Pred/MTX/VCR ADM/EDX MMC/VBL	61
Franciosi	56	Breast	CDDP-VP16	39
Boogerd	20	Breast	EDX/5FU/MTX 5FU/ADM/EDX	76
Kristensen	116	SCLC	Epipodophyllotoxin + CDDP or CBDCA	76
Franciosi	43	NSCLC	CDDP-VP16	30
Boogerd	13	NSCLC	Teniposide	23
Minotti	23	NSCLC	Teniposide-CDDP	35
Crino	47	NSCLC	CDDP-Gemcitabine MMC-Ifo-CDDP	40

NSCLC, non-small cell lung cancer; SCLC, small cell lung cancer; EDX, cyclophosphamide; 5FU, 5-fluorouracil; Pred, prednisone; MTX, methotrexate; VCR, vincristine; ADM, doxorubicine; VBL, vinblastine; VP-16, etoposide; MMC, mitomycin C; CDDP, cisplatin; CBDCA, carboplatin; Ifo, ifosfamide.

solid tumors have shown a substantial equivalence of responsiveness of cranial and extracranial disease. Therefore, chemotherapy can be considered as first option in patients with asymptomatic brain metastases.

Recent advantages in the field of radiotherapy and neurosurgery suggest that, for selected patients, surgery or stereotaxic radiotherapy may be an effective treatment, and, in many cases, a multidisciplinary approach is preferable (Table 8.5).

Several factors interfere with the therapeutic strategy, such as histology of the primary tumor, patient compliance, localization, size and number of brain metastases and outcome of extracranial disease. Generally, surgery or stereo-taxic radiotherapy followed by whole brain radiotherapy is indicated in

Table 8.5 Management of patients with brain metastases

Extracranial disease	Brain metastases	Symptoms	Therapy
Controlled	Single	Absent	Surgery or radiosurgery ± WBRT
		Present	Surgery or radiosurgery ± WBRT
	Multiple	Absent	Chemotherapy or WBRT
		Present	WBRT
Uncontrolled	Single	Absent	Chemotherapy or radiosurgery
		Present	WBRT or radiosurgery
	Multiple	Absent	Chemotherapy or WBRT
		Present	WBRT

WBRT, whole brain radiotherapy.

patients with controlled extracranial disease and good performance status presenting an isolated brain metastasis.

Adding chemotherapy in this subset of patients remains controversial and depends on primary tumor histology and other factors, such as physician cultural biases in evaluating risk/benefit ratio.

Another important issue is the treatment of brain micrometastases. Effectiveness of chemotherapy on micrometastatic brain disease is not clear, and the role of prophylactic cranial irradiation has been well defined only in small cell lung cancer.

Further reading

Auperin A, Arriagada R, Pignon JM et al: Prophylactic cranial irradiation for patients with small-cell lung cancer in complete remission. Prophylactic Cranial Irradiation Overview Collaborative Group. N Engl J Med 1999; 341: 476–84.

Boogerd W, Dalesio O, Bais EM, van der Sande JJ: Response of brain metastases from breast cancer to systemic chemotherapy. Cancer 1992; 69: 972–80.

Clinical practice guidelines for the treatment of unresectable non-small-cell lung cancer. J Clin Oncol 1997; 15:2996–3018.

Patchell RA, Tibbs PA, Walsh JW et al: A randomized trial of surgery in the treatment of single metastases to the brain. N Engl J Med 1990; 322: 494–500.

9 Renal failure and urologic emergencies in cancer patients

S Jezdic, S Jelic
Institute of Oncology and Radiology of Serbia, Serbia and Montenegro

Introduction

Renal failure and urologic emergencies in cancer patients may be caused by disease progression, treatment or unrelated medical conditions. Initial evaluation of symptoms leads to diagnosis and initial management but for definitive treatment referral to a nephrologic and urologic department may be necessary.

Renal failure

Introduction

Renal failure is defined as a loss of renal function and concentrating ability. It is characterized by the presence of progressive uremia; water and electrolyte imbalance; metabolic acidosis; and oliguria rather than anuria, which are caused by acute (acute renal failure) or prolonged (chronic renal failure) decreases in the glomerular filtration rate.

In cancer patients all types of acute renal failure (prerenal, renal and postrenal) may be present. Each type is clinically defined by an initial, maintenance and recovery phase.

Etiology

Prerenal and renal kidney failure

Causes of prerenal and renal insufficiency are given in Tables 9.1 and Table 9.2.

Chemotherapy

Certain chemotherapeutics agents are nephrotoxic (Table 9.3) and there are agents that may be used to protect the kidney. The Food and Drug

Table 9.1 Prerenal causes of acute kidney failure

Type of disturbance	Conditions
Hypovolemia	Hemorrhage, emesis, diarrhea, nasogastric suction, enterostoma, drainage, diuretics, osmotic diuresis, peritonitis, surgical procedures
Minute volume decrease	Myocardial infarction, congestive heart failure, pericardial tamponade, pulmonary embolism
Systemic vasodilatation	Sepsis, antihypertensive drugs, anesthetics, anaphylaxis
Renal vasoconstriction	Hypercalcemia
Renal hypoperfusion with autoregulation dysfunction	Drugs
Hyperviscosity syndrome	Multiple myeloma, macroglobulinemia, polycythemia

Table 9.2 Renal causes of acute kidney failure

Type of injury	Conditions
Glomerular disease	Radiation nephritis, immune complex disease
Interstitial nephritis	Infections, infiltrations (lymphoma, leukemia)
Acute tubular necrosis	Chemotherapy toxicity (Table 9.3)
Intratubular obstruction	Multiple myeloma
Renovascular compression	Compression by tumor or metastasis

Administration (FDA) has approved amifostine to prevent the nephrotoxicity associated with repeated administration of cisplatin in patients with advanced ovarian and non-small cell lung cancer. There is no suggestion that effectiveness of cisplatin-based chemotherapy can be altered by amifostine in these settings. In other settings, where chemotherapy can produce a significant survival advantage or cure, there are only limited data on the effects of amifostine on the efficacy of chemotherapy and amifostine should not be administered except in the context of clinical trials.

Table 9.3 Cytotoxic drugs and type of related nephrotoxicity, clinical features and treatment measures

Cytotoxic agent	Type of renal injury	Clinical features	Treatment	Preventive measures
Cisplatin	Necrosis of proximal convoluted tubules	Renal tubular acidosis	• Withdrawal of drug • Dialysis • Replacement of HCO_3, PO_4, Mg^{2+}	• Hydration with mannitol • Diuretics administration* • Dose adjustment based on creatinine clearance • Avoidance of other nephrotoxic drugs
Carboplatin	Tubular	Magnesium wasting	• Withdrawal of drug • Dialysis if necessary	• GFR-based dosing to achieve a targeted area under the curve (AUC) • Avoidance of nephrotoxicity drugs
Mitomycin C	Vascular lesions	Hemolytic uremic syndrome (HUS)	• Drug withdrawal • Dialysis	• Stop drug at cumulative dose of 50 mg/m^2
Methotrexate	Necrosis of convoluted tubules	Oliguria	• High-dose leucovorin based on plasma methotrexate level • Urine alkalinization	• Ensuring adequate hydration • Alkalinizing urine to pH 7 or higher • Avoidance of other nephrotoxic drugs

Table 9.3 Continued

Cytotoxic agent	Type of renal injury	Clinical features	Treatment	Preventive measures
Interleukin-2	Capillary leak syndrome	Oliguria and hypotension	• Drug withdrawal • Hydration	• Dopamine and fluids
Ifosfamide	Acute tubular necrosis	Oliguria	• Supportive dialysis	• See Table 9.4
Gemcitabine	Vascular lesions	HUS	• Gemcitabine discontinuation • Dialysis	
Nitrosoureas (lomustine, carmustine)	Interstitial nephritis		• Dialysis	• Stop carmustine at cumulative dose of 1200 mg/m^2

* Conflicting reports exist regarding usage of furosemide (frusemide); GFR: glomerular filtration rate.

Radiotherapy

Radiotherapy may also cause nephrotoxicity and the kidney is an important dose-limiting organ during radiation. Glomerular function starts to decrease at 15 Gy and function is completely lost at radiation doses of 25–30 Gy. Radiosensitizers such as cisplatin tend to decrease normal tissue tolerance. Symptoms are rarely seen acutely within 6 months of treatment. Subacute symptoms are seen 6–12 months after radiotherapy.

Long-term nephrotoxicity related to total-body irradiation in the bone marrow transplantation setting is associated with symptoms caused by subendothelial widening of the basal membrane, endothelial cell dropout, glomerular arteriolar intimal thickening and tubular atrophy.

Postrenal kidney failure

Urinary obstruction can occur in the upper or lower urinary tract:

- Upper urinary tract obstruction in cancer patients of one or both urethers can be caused by:
  - direct tumor invasion
  - compression or encasement from metastatic retroperitoneal or pelvic lymph nodes
  - direct metastasis to the ureter.
- Malignant tumors that can be a source of ureteral obstruction are cervical, bladder, prostate, gastrointestinal, breast and testicular cancer, lymphoma and other tumors.
- Additionally, retroperitoneal fibrosis due to specific treatment may be a source of ureteral compression.
- Lower urinary tract obstruction may be caused by:
  - mechanical factors due to cancer
  - neurophysiologic factors due to cancer
  - treatment
  - pre-existing benign conditions.
- Complete bladder outlet obstruction can lead to bilateral hydroureteronephrosis with renal failure. Distal outlet obstructions are caused by locally advanced tumors that invade the urethra or primary urethral, prostate or bladder tumors.

Evaluation

Symptoms

Patients with renal insufficiency may complain of fatigue, dyspnea, anorexia and nausea and vomiting. Symptoms of acute ureteral obstruction are flank pain and colics. Acute urine retention and bladder outlet obstruction are presented with symptoms of dysuria, frequency and nycturia.

Examination

Clinical examination may show palpebral or peripheral edema, tachypnea, tachycardia, and lumbar pain. Pathologically, acute urinary tract obstruction results in increased central renal pressure and dilatation of the ureter. On the ultrasonography examination, this is reflected in increased size of the kidney. With persistent and progressive obstructive uropathy, irreversible injury finally manifests itself with renal cortical atrophy.

Glomerular filtration rate

The most common renal function abnormality as a side effect of cytotoxic therapy is decline in glomerular filtration rate (GFR). Creatinine clearance is the most frequent parameter used for GFR estimation. The Cockroft–Gault formula is most commonly used for this purpose. Although it has significant limitations for estimating creatinine clearance from serum creatinine level alone, it is widely applied in clinical oncology. The wide fluctuations in weight that occur in cancer patients undergoing chemotherapy require that patients be weighed before each cycle of chemotherapy and doses adjusted on the basis of weight changes. The Cockroft–Gault formula is

$$\frac{(140 - age) \times Weight\ (kg)}{72 \times Serum\ creatinine\ (mg/dl)} \quad (\times 0.85\ for\ women)$$

The serum creatinine level is mostly determined in $\mu mol/L$, so the following formula should be used:

$$\frac{(140 - age) \times Weight\ (kg)}{0.81 \times Serum\ creatinine\ (\mu mol/L)}$$

The Cockroft–Gault formula has been recommended by the FDA guidelines for dose adjustments in renal impairment. More recently, a more accurate formula for estimation of GFR has been developed and validated for drug disposition in patients with renal impairment. This formula estimates body surface area – indexed GFR.

Laboratory analysis

Acute and chronic bilateral obstruction are presented with uremia. The first indication of obstructive uropathy is frequently a rising serum creatinine level and, in addition, the blood urea level.

Urinary indices

The differential diagnosis of prerenal and renal insufficiency can be made by urinary indices:

Fractional excretion of sodium (FE_{Na}) = (Sodium excretion × 100)/(total filtered load)

with   Sodium excretion = (Urine sodium)/(Serum sodium)

and   Total load = (Urine creatinine)/(Serum creatinine)

$$FE_{Na} = (u_{Na} \times s_{Cr} \times 100)/(s_{Na} \times u_{Cr})$$

If FE_{Na} <1%: prerenal insufficiency

If FE_{Na} >2%: renal insufficiency

For urine sodium:

     <30 mEq/L: prerenal insufficiency

     >30 mEq/L: renal insufficiency

Urinalysis

Urine should be checked on proteinuria, hematuria and casts.

Echography

Echography is the examination of choice to diagnose obstructive uropathy in patients with renal insufficiency.

Imaging

Chronic unilateral obstruction is often diagnosed incidentally on imaging studies of the upper abdomen as hydronephrosis with renal cortical atrophy. Diagnostic studies can be made by intravenous urography, computed tomography (CT), renal ultrasonography, retrograde pyelography, radionuclide renography and endourethral ultrasonography.

Treatment of acute renal failure

Preventive measures

Management of medications

- Assess medications for toxicity:
    - check drug levels
    - adjust dosages for renal function.
- Stop nephrotoxic drugs:
    - nonsteroidal anti-inflammatory drugs (NSAIDs)
    - angiotensin-converting enzyme (ACE) inhibitors
    - aminoglycosides
    - avoid repeating radiocontrast material
    - avoid high-dose diuretics in critically ill patients
    - avoid nephrotoxic chemotherapeutics.

Conservative treatment

Management of volume status

- Normal volume status:
    - limit fluid intake to urine output + 300–500 ml/day
    - limit sodium intake to 2 g/day.
- Volume overload:
    - limit fluid intake to less than urine output
    - limit sodium intake to less than 2 g/day
    - consider loop diuretic
    - consider dialysis.
- Volume depletion:
    - restore volume with isotonic saline
    - limit intake to urine output + 300–500 ml/day
    - limit sodium intake to 2 g/day.

Management of potassium

- Hyperkalemia:
    - look for potassium source
    - eliminate parenteral potassium
    - reduce dietary potassium intake <50 mEq/day
    - consider potassium-binding resin (e.g. sodium polystyrene sulfonate (Kayexalate®))
    - consider dialysis.
- Normokalemia:
    - limit potassium intake to 50 mEq/day.

Management of acid–base status

- Acidemia:
  - look for cause of acidosis
  - reduce protein intake to 0.6 g/kg/day
  - consider oral bicarbonate or isotonic intravenous (IV) bicarbonate
  - consider dialysis.
- Normal pH:
  - limit protein intake to 0.8 g/kg/day.

Nutritional intake

- Maintain 30–50 kcal/kg/day.

Management of uremia

- Absent:
  - limit protein intake to 0.9 g/kg/day.
- Present:
  - reduce protein to 0.6 g/kg/day
  - check for gastrointestinal bleeding.

Dialysis

In case of severe fluid and electrolyte disturbances, dialysis is indicated:

- blood urea nitrogen >150 mg/dl
- serum creatinine >10 g/dl
- uremic symptoms.

Obstructive nephropathy

- Ureteral decompression should be undertaken and is followed by diuresis and renal function normalization. In the absence of significant atrophy, the obstructed kidney will most likely regain significant function and CT- or ultrasound-guided percutaneous nephrostomy should be considered with monitoring of renal function, CT and renal ultrasound, urine cultures and replacement of stent or tube every 4–6 months.
- Tubular defects can result in a brisk postobstructive diuresis. Replacement of fluid and electrolytes is important until normal renal function returns.
- Small atrophic kidneys due to long-standing obstructive uropathy frequently do not benefit from placement of Foley catheters or suprapubic tubes.
- Suprapubic tube placement in urothelial malignancies with curative intent is contraindicated because it violates the normal anatomic barriers and

increases the probability of regional spread of the disease. Percutaneous nephrostomies are used more frequently than surgically constructed urinary diversion in such circumstances.

Cystitis

Introduction

Symptomatic cystitis is a bladder irritation presented by suprapubic discomfort, frequency, dysuria, urgency and severe manifestations of urge incontinence and hematuria.

Etiology

The etiology related to the oncologic circumstances may be:

- toxic effects of cytotoxic drugs (Table 9.3)
- radiotherapy
- thrombocytopenia accompanied with bleeding
- infection in neutropenic settings
- malignancy.

Treatment

Chemical cystitis

Alkylating agents (oxazaphosphorines, cyclophosphamide and ifosfamide) have cumulative and dose-dependent urothelial toxic effects. Urinary excretion of their metabolites is a major source of urothelial toxicity.

Hemorrhagic cystitis can be managed by:

- stopping, reducing or replacing the drug
- hydration and enhanced diuresis in order to dilute the metabolites in the urine
- mesna (Uromitexan®) is recommended to decrease the incidence of oxazaphosphorine-associated urothelial toxicity (Table 9.4).

The first dose of mesna is administered intravenously, at a dose equal to 20% of the total daily ifosfamide dose, followed by mesna tablets given orally in a dosage equal to 40% of the ifosfamide dose at 2 and 6 hours after each dose of ifosfamide. The total daily dose of mesna is 100% of the ifosfamide dose. In case of vomiting within 2 hours of taking oral mesna, repetition of the dose or receiving IV mesna is indicated.

Table 9.4 *Recommendation for mesna usage*

Oxazaphosphorines schedule	Recommended dose of mesna
Standard dose ifosfamide* – less than 2 g/m²/day (short infusion)	60% of the total daily dose of ifosfamide, administered as 3 bolus doses (15 minutes before, 4 and 8 hours after administration of each dose of ifosfamide)
Standard dose ifosfamide – less than 2 g/m²/day (continuous infusion)	Bolus dose equal to 20% of the total ifosfamide dose followed by a continuous infusion of mesna equal to 40% of the ifosfamide dose, continuing for 12–24 hours after completion of the ifosfamide infusion
High-dose ifosfamide – dose in excess of 2.5 g/m²/day	• The efficacy of mesna for urothelial protection has not been established • More frequent and prolonged mesna dosage regimens may be necessary
High-dose cyclophosphamide in the setting of stem-cell transplantation	Mesna plus saline diuresis

* Mesna administration by the oral route has been also approved by the FDA.

Radiation cystitis

Patients undergoing radiotherapy for cervical, uterine, bladder, rectal and prostate cancer have an enhanced risk of direct or incidental urothelial damage especially in settings of concomitant urinary infection, high-dose radiotherapy or prior surgery in the area.

After an acute inflammatory response, in a further course patients can develop symptoms that are dose-dependent and present with bladder ulcers and fibrosis and ureteral strictures. These patients are at increased risk of developing transitional cell carcinoma of the bladder.

Thrombocytopenia accompanied with bleeding

Platelet concentrates are used.

Acute or chronic bacterial cystitis

Acute or chronic bacterial cystitis is usually not accompanied with fever or an elevated leukocyte count. Urinary tract infections are mainly ascending, with an indwelling bladder catheter as the principal port of entry. Ascending invasion of the renal epithelium (acute pyelonephritis) may cause infiltrates in the kidneys associated with fever, flank pain, bacteremia and an elevated leukocyte count.

A diagnostic approach to an urinary tract infection is urine and blood culture and renal imaging. Complications may be stone formation, renal cortical abscess, renal carbuncle, emphysematous pyelonephritis and urinary sepsis. Urinary sepsis should be specially emphasized as an oncologic emergency in neutropenic setting.

Viral hemorrhagic cystitis

Viral agents (adenovirus type 11, HIV) may cause late-onset hemorrhagic cystitis in bone marrow recipients.

Acute epididymitis or prostatitis

When urethral or bladder pathogens pass the vas deferens and prostate ducts, they cause acute epididymitis or prostatitis. Patients present with fever and local pain that require empiric antibiotic treatment for 10–14 days and measures such as scrotal elevation, warm baths and anti-inflammatory agents. An abscess may develop that requires emergent surgical drainage.

Periurethral abscess

A periurethral abscess is a life-threatening infection of the male urethra and periurethral tissues (perineal and scrotal) and should be differentiated from tissue edema, follicular and perirectal abscess, Fournier's gangrene and penile or urethral cancer. Emergent debridement, suprapubic drainage of urine and broad-spectrum antibiotics are treatment options, together with preventive measures of recurrence.

Bladder hemorrhage

In case of gross hematuria and clotting, the patient may develop urine retention. It is urgent to re-establish urine outflow by inserting a large-diameter, multiple-hole urethral catheter and to perform saline lavage and clot evacuation. If lavage is not effective, endoscopic clot evacuation under anesthesia should be performed.

If diffuse bleeding continues, intravesical instillation of a hemostatic agent is indicated. Persistent bladder hemorrhage despite conservative measures may necessitate open cystectomy with bladder packing, cutaneous ureterostomy and embolization of the artery or cystectomy with urinary diversion.

Priapism

Priapism is a painful erection that is not associated with sexual stimulation and is a medical emergency. In cancer patients, priapism may be due to primary malignancy (hematologic diseases), medication intake and tumor infiltration or metastases from penile, prostate, bladder and kidney cancer. Treatment of malignant priapism consists of analgesia for pain relief and treatment of the underlying malignancy.

Further reading

Brady HR, Brenner BM, Lieberthal W: Acute renal failure. In: Brenner B et al (eds), The Kidney. Philadelphia: WB Saunders, 1996: 1200–38.

Cockroft DW, Gault MH: Prediction of creatinine clearance from serum creatinine. Nephron 1976; 16: 31–41.

Lesesne JB, Rothschild NO, Erickson B et al: Cancer-associated hemolytic-uremic syndrome: analysis of 85 cases from a national registry. J Clin Onc 1989; 7: 781–9.

Lokich J, Anderson N: Carboplatin versus cisplatin in solid tumors: an analysis of the literature. Ann Onc 1998; 9: 13–21.

Nackaerts K, Daenen N, Vansteenkiste J et al: Hemolytic-uremic syndrome caused by gemcitabine. Ann Oncol 1998; 9: 1355.

Russo P: Urologic emergencies. In: De Vita V, Hellman S, Rosenberg SA (eds), Cancer Principles and Practice of Oncology, 5th edn. Philadelphia: Lippincott-Raven, 1997: 2512–22.

Schiffer AC, Anderson AK, Bennett LC et al: Platelet transfusion for patients with cancer: Clinical Practice Guidelines of the American Society of Clinical Oncology. J Clin Onc 2001; 19: 1519–38.

Schuchter LM, Hensley ML, Meropol NJ, Winer EP: 2002 Update of Recommendations for the Use of Chemotherapy and Radiotherapy Protectants: Clinical Practice Guidelines of the American Society of Clinical Oncology. J Clin Onc 2002; 20: 2895–903.

Takimoto CH, Remick SC, Sharma S et al: A dose escalating and pharmacological study of oxaliplatin in adult cancer patients with impaired renal function: a National Cancer Institute Organ Dysfunction Group study. J Clin Onc 2003; 21: 2664–72.

10 Hypercalcemia

S Rottey, S Van Belle
Medical Oncology, University Hospital Gent, Belgium

Introduction

Hypercalcemia is the most frequent metabolic complication of cancer, with its reported incidence ranging from 15–20 per 100 000 persons. Apparently, patients suffering from breast cancer, multiple myeloma, non-small cell lung cancer and hypernephroma seem most at risk for developing hypercalcemia.

Etiology

The current concept of cancer-related hypercalcemia is that both in the presence or absence of tumor-induced bone destruction, circulating factors secreted by the malignant cells can be held responsible.

Parathyroid hormone (parathormone or PTH) and parathyroid hormone-related protein (PTHrp)

Apart from parathyroid carcinoma, tumors producing PTH are rare. In contrast, PTHrp is the most common cause of cancer-related hypercalcemia. PTHrp is homologous for 8 of the 13 amino-terminal amino acids, resulting in the capability of binding the PTH receptor. In physiological conditions, PTHrp is a paracrine factor, not acting via the systemic circulation. When overproduction in tumor cells occurs, the hormone acts systemically, stimulating intestinal calcium uptake, tubular calcium reabsorption and bone metabolism.

Vitamin D_3

In patients with Hodgkin's disease, non-Hodgkin's lymphoma and multiple myeloma elevated $1,25\text{-}(OH)_2$ vitamin D_3 levels have been observed. This has been hypothesized to be related to an increase of 1-alpha hydroxylase activity in tumor cells, causing accelerated transition from 25-OH to $1,25\text{-}(OH)_2$ vitamin D_3. Whether this finding should be considered causal for the observed hypercalcemia is a point of discussion.

Prostaglandins

Prostaglandins may play a local role in cancer-related osteolysis but are rarely implicated in hypercalcemia of malignancy.

Cytokines

Transforming growth factor is secreted by many cancer cells in an autocrine way. Because of partial amino acid homology, it may stimulate the epidermal growth factor (EGF) receptor, inducing enhanced bone resorption. Other growth factors – e.g. interleukins IL-1 and IL-6 and tumor necrosis factor (TNF) induce bone resorption in vitro, but their clinical significance has not been shown in vivo. These factors act in the proximity of tumor cells, transforming infiltrating macrophages into osteoclasts, and thus generating lytic lesions.

Differential diagnosis

It should be kept in mind that, although numerous diseases (Box 10.1) can cause hypercalcemia, most frequent amongst these are hyperparathyroidism and malignancy. If hypercalcemia occurs in a hospitalized patient, there is a 65% likelihood that it is associated with malignancy.

Evaluation

A standardized approach to the diagnosis of hypercalcemia usually helps to elucidate the cause quickly (Figure 10.1).

- Early manifestations of hypercalcemia can be very insidious, including fatigue, muscle weakness, depression, vague abdominal pain, constipation and anorexia. They can be easily mistaken for manifestations of the underlying malignant disease.
- Besides nonspecific gastrointestinal manifestations, hypercalcemia can sporadically cause pancreatitis and a predisposition to peptic ulcers.
- The renal complications can be subdivided into acute and chronic complications. An acute rise in calcemia causes renal vasoconstriction and natriuresis-induced volume contraction, leading to a reversible fall in glomerular filtration. Long-lasting hypercalcemia induces concentrating defects, leading to nephrogenic diabetes insipidus. Also, renal tubular acidosis, nephrolithiasis and chronic renal insufficiency are observed.
- The degree of neuropsychiatric disturbances varies with calcium concentrations, starting with slight cognitive dysfunction and anxiety with

Cancer
- PTHrp-related
- Other circulating factors

Endocrine and metabolic disease
- Familial hypocalciuric hypercalcemia
- Exogenous thyroid hormone administration
- Primary hyperparathyroidism
- Addison's disease
- Immobilization

Infection and granulomatosis
- Tuberculosis
- HIV
- Sarcoidosis
- Berylliosis
- Coccidioidomycosis

Diet and drugs
- Exogenous vitamin D
- Exogenous vitamin A
- Lithium
- Calcium supplements
- Milk-alkali syndrome
- Thiazide and diuretics

moderate hypercalcemia and evolving into hallucinations, psychosis, somnolence and coma with high calcemia.
- Cardiovascular complications are a tendency towards hypertension and accelerated calcium deposition in endothelial structures.
- Urinary calcium excretion is usually high normal or elevated. In rare cases this parameter is low: milk-alkali syndrome, use of thiazide diuretics and familial hypocalciuric hypercalcemia.

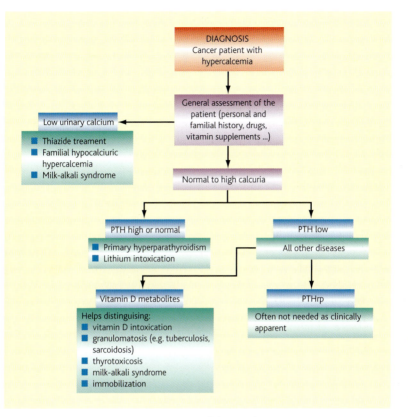

Figure 10.1 Diagnosis of a cancer patient with hypercalcemia

- Phosphatemia is usually low in humoral hypercalcemia of malignancy and hyperparathyroidism, but is often elevated in metastatic bone disease.
- Serum PTH levels: in case of primary hyperparathyroidism and of lithium intoxication, intact PTH is expected to be inappropriately normal or high. All other causes of hypercalcemia are associated with low (suppressed) PTH.
- Measurement of PTHrp may be performed if patients are thought to have humoral hypercalcemia of malignancy. However, since most of these patients have advanced disease, this parameter is seldom useful because of the apparent clinical correlation with the underlying disease.

- Vitamin D metabolites can be determined if no malignancy is obvious and if neither PTH nor PTHrp are elevated.

Treatment

The ultimate treatment of hypercalcemia of malignancy is curing the malignancy. More often than not, this is not feasible since most patients already have metastatic disease at the time of appearance of hypercalcemia (Box 10.2).

Limiting oral calcium intake

This is discouraged, since its effect is highly limited.

Increasing urinary calcium excretion

Intravenous saline

Intravenous saline induces volume expansion, inhibiting sodium reabsorption in the proximal tubule. As proximal calcium reabsorption is a passive process, dependent on the gradient established by sodium reabsorption, calciuria increases. Theoretically, blocking the Na/K/Cl carrier in Henle's loop by using diuretics (e.g. furosemide (frusemide)) could enhance calciuria. However, in

Box 10.2 Treatment options in hypercalcemia

General measures
- Reduce immobilization
- Stop or limit drugs that inhibit renal calcium excretion: e.g. thiazide diuretics
- Stop or limit drugs that lower renal perfusion: e.g. nonsteroidal anti-inflammatory drugs (NSAIDs), angiotensin-converting enzyme (ACE)-inhibitors, angiotensin II receptor blockers
- Stop supplementary intake of vitamins D, A and other retinoids: e.g. multivitamin preparations

Specific measures
- Increase urinary calcium excretion: saline, furosemide (frusemide)
- Inhibit bone resorption: bisphosphonates, gallium nitrate, calcitonin, corticosteroids

vivo, this calciuretic effect is counteracted by volume contraction induced by the diuretic. It should be stressed that the above-mentioned measures are seldom enough to render patients normocalcemic (20% of patients with a calcemia >12 mg/dl become normocalcemic after a single course of therapy), but adequate hydration is a cornerstone in the treatment.

Inhibition of bone resorption

Bisphosphonates

Bisphosphonates are nonhydrolyzable analogs of inorganic pyrophosphate. Their mechanism of action is absorption to the surface of bone hydroxyapatite, thus inhibiting calcium release by interfering with the osteoclast metabolic activity. As these agents are relatively non-toxic – adverse events: pyrexia, hypophosphatemia and the mild gastrointestinal distress – and more potent than other drugs inhibiting bone resorption, they have become one of the essential measures in the treatment of cancer-induced hypercalcemia. It should be remembered that their maximum effect occurs only after 2–4 days, necessitating other treatment measures with swifter action. Because of the superiority of later-generation bisphosphonates over those of the first generation (e.g. etidronate, clodronate), these first-generation products will not be discussed.

Pamidronate was until recently the agent of choice, taking into account its augmented potency and its longer action period (response often sustained for 2–4 weeks). The maximum calcium response occurs at 90 mg intravenously, but some clinicians adjust their dosage to the degree of hypercalcemia. The minimum dosage interval is weekly, but in practice this is every 2–4 weeks. A less favorable response is seen in patients with PTHrp-induced hypercalcemia, who respond better to gallium citrate.

Zoledronate has become the treatment of choice for cancer-induced hypercalcemia because of its still higher potency (88% and 70% of the patients achieve normocalcemia after single-dose treatment with zoledronate and pamidronate, respectively) and significantly shorter infusion period (15 minutes). Furthermore, the duration of calcium control increases to 1–1.5 months. Renal toxicity and osteonecrosis have been reported.

Risedronate is a third-generation product that can be given orally. It is still under evaluation in the indication of hypercalcemia.

Gallium nitrate

Gallium inhibits osteoclastic bone resorption via inhibition of an ATPase-dependent proton pump on the osteoclast ruffled membrane. Its effect is independent of the presence of circulating PTHrp. It has been reported to be more effective in standard doses than pamidronate (72% versus 59% normocalcemia). The disadvantages are nephrotoxicity and the prolonged (5 days) need of continuous intravenous infusion. Being a relatively new treatment method, it is expected that gallium will be used more frequently in the near future.

Calcitonin

Calcitonin decreases bone resorption and also increases the urinary clearance of calcium. It should be administered intramuscularly or subcutaneously every 12 hours. It is a relatively weak compound (lowering of calcemia by 1–2 mg/dl), but its main advantage is that it acts rapidly (within 6 hours). However, its effect is limited to the first 24 hours. Apart from gastrointestinal discomfort and hypersensitivity, it has limited side effects. Hence, it is the ideal treatment of choice immediately after the diagnosis to bridge the time of action of other agents (e.g. bisphosphonates).

Calcium removal/chelation

- Sodium EDTA (ethylenediaminetetraacetic acid) and intravenous phosphate can form complexes with ionized calcium, after which these are cleared from circulation. They act immediately, but are toxic: they are replaced by the above-mentioned agents.
- Dialysis is the ultimate rescue treatment in patients with uncontrollable or severe hypercalcemia. It can be considered when hypercalcemia is accompanied by renal failure.

Corticosteroids

Corticosteroids inhibit osteoclast-mediated bone resorption in vitro and decrease gastrointestinal calcium uptake. These drugs should only be prescribed in patients with malignancies susceptible to steroids (e.g. myeloma, lymphoma, leukemia and occasionally breast cancer). Doses of methylprednisolone range from 15–30 mg/day in breast cancer to 40–100 mg/day in hematologic diseases.

The treatment decision tree (Figure 10.1) is a proposition to initiate adequate treatment rapidly in cancer patients, and is tailored to the clinical situation.

Further reading

Bockman R: The effects of gallium nitrate on bone resorption. Semin Oncol 2003; 30(2 Suppl 5): 5–12.

Carano A, Teitelbaum SL, Konsek JD et al: Bisphosphonates directly inhibit the bone resorption activity of isolated avian osteoclasts in vitro. J Clin Invest 1990; 85: 456–61.

Gardner EC Jr, Hersh T: Primary hyperparathyroidism and the gastrointestinal tract. South Med J 1981; 74: 197–9.

Gurney H, Grill V, Martin TJ: Parathyroid hormone-related protein and response to pamidronate in tumor-induced hypercalcaemia. Lancet 1993; 341: 1611–13.

Heath H 3d: Clinical spectrum of primary hyperparathyroidism: evolution with changes in medical practice and technology. J Bone Miner Res 1991; 6(Suppl 2): S63.

Major P, Lortholary A, Hon J et al: Zoledronic acid is superior to pamidronate in the treatment of hypercalcemia of malignancy: a pooled analysis of two randomized, controlled clinical trials. J Clin Oncol 2001; 19: 558–67.

Nussbaum SR, Younger J, Vandepol CJ et al: Single-dose intravenous therapy with pamidronate for the treatment of hypercalcemia of malignancy: comparison of 30-, 60-, and 90-mg dosages. Am J Med 1993; 95:297–304.

Quinn JM, Matsumura Y, Tarin D et al: Cellular and hormonal mechanisms associated with malignant bone resorption. Lab Invest 1994; 71: 465–71.

Raue F: Epidemiological aspects of hypercalcemia of malignancy. Recent Results Cancer Res 1994; 137: 99–106.

Warrell RP Jr: Metabolic emergencies. In: De Vita V, Hellman S, Rosenberg SA (eds), Cancer: Principles and Practice of Oncology. Philadelphia: Lippincott-Raven, 1997: 2486–93.

Wysolmerski JJ, Broadus AE: Hypercalcemia of malignancy: the central role of parathyroid hormone-related protein. Annu Rev Med 1994; 45: 189–200.

11 Acute tumor lysis syndrome

DM Kraemer, K Wilms
University of Würzburg, Germany

Introduction

Rapid lysis of malignant cells leads to a release of cellular metabolites, especially uric acid and intracellular ions, exceeding the excretory capacity of the kidneys. Life-threatening disturbances of metabolism and electrolyte balance might follow. Acute tumor lysis syndrome (ATLS) depends on:

- tumor-associated factors, such as size and grading
- patient-associated factors, such as impaired renal function
- therapy-related factors.

Rapid cell lysis leads to a release of large amounts of nucleic acids, potassium and phosphate. Nucleic acids consist of purines, which are metabolized via xanthine oxidase to hypoxanthine, xanthine and finally uric acid. If the concentration of uric acid increases and the pH decreases, uric acid precipitates in kidney tubules. Renal impairment follows, which may lead to acidosis, further enhancing precipitation of uric acid.

In addition to uric acid, potassium ions are released during rapid cell lysis. This effect can be detected as early as 6 hours after the start of chemotherapy. If renal function is impaired because of precipitated uric acid, potassium ions cannot be eliminated.

Also, phosphate is released following lysis of malignant cells. For example, lymphoblasts contain four times more phosphate than lymphocytes. The serum phosphate level increases 24 hours after cell lysis. If the pH is high, phosphate is precipitated with calcium, as calcium phosphate which can be found in different tissues but especially in the renal parenchyma. Nephrocalcinosis might develop, leading to further renal impairment. Serum calcium levels decrease.

Etiology

Chemotherapy

Patients diagnosed with rapidly proliferating malignancies (aggressive lymphomas, especially Burkitt's lymphoma, acute lymphoblastic or myeloid leukemia or even multiple myeloma) are at high risk of developing a tumor lysis syndrome. The syndrome occurs most often in children, since they frequently suffer from very aggressive types of cancer.

Most often, ATLS occurs during induction chemotherapy. In rare cases, ATLS is diagnosed in solid tumors, as seminoma or medulloblastoma.

Other anticancer treatments

ATLS has also been described during radiation therapy, treatment with corticosteroids or monoclonal antibodies.

Nephrotoxic drugs

The use of nephrotoxic drugs such as aminoglycosides or nonsteroidal antiphlogistics might increase renal dysfunction. Additionally, obstruction of the ureter by the malignant tumor might intensify renal impairment.

Evaluation

Symptoms

Patients might show symptoms of hypocalcemia as confusion, tetany, muscle cramps or cardiac arrhythmia. Bradycardia, arrhythmia and circulatory collapse might be the consequence. Patients with hyperkalemia might suffer from weakness of muscles or lethargy.

Risk factors

High risk factors for developing ATLS (Box 11.1):

- elevated lactate dehydrogenase > 1000 U/L
- leukocytes >50 000/μl
- uric acid >6.5 mg/dl
- bulky disease
- impaired renal function with elevated creatinine
- initial dehydration.

Clinical signs

Clinically significant ATLS is characterized by one of the following parameters occurring during the first 4 days of therapy:

- potassium >6 mmol/L (discriminate from an artifact due to slow drawing of blood!)
- creatinine >2.4 mg/dl
- calcium <6 mg/dl
- life-threatening arrhythmia
- increase of more than 25% of phosphate, uric acid or urea in comparison to the baseline values.

Disseminated intravascular coagulopathy

Sometimes ATLS is associated with disseminated intravascular coagulopathy (DIC).

Electrocardiogram

The electrocardiogram (ECG) shows elevated T waves and widening of QRS complexes.

Prevention and treatment

Prevention of ATLS

The most important factors are to acknowledge the risk of ATLS and to prevent its development. Patients with risk factors should receive induction therapy in an inpatient setting on a hematology ward.

- Prophylactic hydration is the most effective preventive therapy. Patients should receive 3–5 L/m^2 of fluid intravenously (half glucose 5%, half NaCl 0.9%).
- Alkalinization of the urine is performed by adding 40 meq of sodium bicarbonate into the glucose solution. The pH of the urine should be controlled (optimal pH between 7 and 7.5).
- Body weight and fluid balance have to be controlled at least twice a day.
- If the patient has risks factors for developing an ATLS, laboratory parameters – uric acid, Na, K, Ca, Mg, phosphate, creatinine, lactate dehydrogenase, international normalized ratio (INR), fibrinogen, blood cell count and glucose – should be controlled at least daily.

Treatment of ATLS

If a clinically relevant ATLS is diagnosed:

- The patient should be transferred to a critical care unit.
- ECG and pulse should be supervised continuously.
- Central venous pressure should be measured every 8 hours.
- Input and output of fluids should be balanced.
- Hydration should be continued with 5 L/m^2.
- Diuresis should be at least 150–200 ml/h. If diuresis is less or the patient is gaining weight under hydration therapy, diuretics, especially furosemide (frusemide), should be added intravenously. Potassium-saving diuretics should be avoided.
- Due to renal impairment, nephrotoxic drugs such as X-ray contrast medium, aminoglycosides and nonsteroidal antiphlogistic drugs should be avoided. Drugs which inhibit excretion of uric acid in the kidney, such as probenecid, aspirin or thiazides should not be used.

Treatment of hyperuricemia in ATLS

■ Allopurinol is the drug of choice to avoid elevation of uric acid. The enzyme xanthine oxidase converts the drug allopurinol into oxypurinol, which inhibits the enzyme itself. Therefore, oxypurinol blocks metabolism of hypoxanthine to uric acid. Figure 11.1 shows the metabolism of purines to uric acid.

Solubility and renal elimination of xanthines are much better than those of uric acid. To prevent ATLS, 10 mg/kg/day of allopurinol, divided into two oral doses, should be administered. If oral application of allopurinol is not possible, allopurinol might be given intravenously. However, the intravenous drug allopurinol is only licensed in the USA.

If renal function is impaired, the dose of allopurinol should be reduced. If the clearance of creatinine is higher than 20 ml/min, 300 mg allopurinol/day is administered. Allopurinol should not be combined with 6-mercatopurine, decumarol, ampicillin or cyclosporine.

If allergic reactions of the skin are visible, urate oxidase or rasburicase should replace allopurinol.

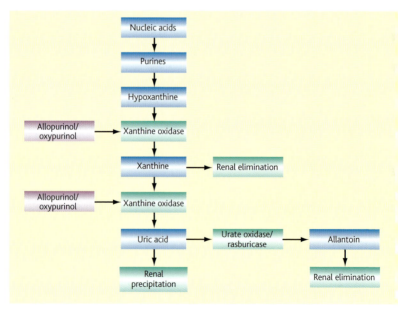

Figure 11.1 Metabolism of nucleic acids

- Urate oxidase metabolizes uric acid into allantoin, which is 10 times more soluble. Nonrecombinant urate oxidase, extracted from the filamentous fungus *Aspergillus flavus,* is marketed as Uricozyme in France and Italy: 4–5% of patients suffer from allergic reactions after application.
- cDNA of the enzyme urate oxidase was cloned from the *Aspergillus flavus* strain and inserted into a yeast vector for expression in *Saccharomyces cerevisiae*. The resulting purified recombinant enzyme rasburicase has recently obtained approval in Europe under the trade name Fasturtec (Elitek in the USA). Fasturtec should be used intravenously at a dose of 0.2 mg/kg/day for 5–7 days, in 50 ml 0.9% NaCl, and infused for 30 min. Reduction of dose because of renal or liver impairment is not necessary. Potential side effects are fever, nausea, vomiting, diarrhea, headache and allergic reactions. In addition to its use in clinically relevant ATLS, rasburicase might be helpful in the treatment of patients with risk factors to prevent ATLS.

Treatment of hyperkalemia in ATLS

If potassium exceeds 5 mmol/L hyperkalemia is diagnosed:

- Mild hyperkalemia (up to potassium levels of 5.5 mmol/L) might be treated with hydration and application of furosemide (frusemide) (Box 11.2).
- In an emergency, potassium levels can be decreased by application of two aerosol doses of beta$_2$-agonists, e.g. fenoterol.
- Application of glucose and insulin decreases potassium levels by pushing potassium ions from extracellular into intracellular compartments: 1 g of glucose might be given per kg of patient body weight per hour, with the application of 1/4 IE insulin (both administered intravenously). For example, a patient with a body weight of 60 kg could receive, during 1 hour,

Box 11.2 *Therapy for ATLS*

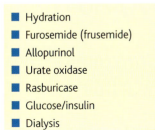

- Hydration
- Furosemide (frusemide)
- Allopurinol
- Urate oxidase
- Rasburicase
- Glucose/insulin
- Dialysis

300 ml of glucose 20% in addition to 15 IE of insulin. Blood glucose and potassium levels should be controlled every 30–60 minutes.

Dialysis in ATLS

If potassium ions exceed 7 mmol/L, the patient is in a life-threatening condition and immediate dialysis should be performed. Other indications for dialysis are potassium > 6 mmol/L under hydration therapy, phosphate >10 mg/dl, urea >150 mg/dl and oliguria or anuria.

Hyperphosphatemia in ATLS

The most effective therapy in hyperphosphatemia is hydration and forced diuresis with furosemide (frusemide). If the patient has no parenteral alimentation, 0.1 g/kg aluminum hydroxide should be administered orally to bind the phosphate in the food. If the phosphate concentration exceeds 10 mg/dl, hemodialysis should be performed.

Hypocalcemia results from precipitation of calcium phosphate based on hyperphosphatemia. Magnesium ions should be determined, because calcium levels cannot be elevated if magnesium ion levels are low. If possible, calcium should be given orally. Application of calcium gluconate might induce cardiac arrhythmia. ECG monitoring is necessary. Intravenous application of calcium gluconate might induce necroses of tissue.

Complications

ATLS is a life-threatening disease, complicated by acute renal failure, malignant arrhythmias, DIC and finally death.

Further reading

Altman A: Acute tumor lysis syndrome. Semin Oncol 2001; 28: 3–8.

Feusner J, Farber MS: Role of intravenous allopurinol in the management of acute tumor lysis syndrome. Semin Oncol 2001; 28: 13–18.

Goldman SC, Holcenberg JS, Finklestein JZ et al: A randomized comparison between rasburicase and allopurinol in children with lymphoma or leukemia at high risk for tumor lysis. Blood 2001; 97: 2998–3003.

Huhn D, Henze G: Tumorlysesyndrom. Stuttgart: Thieme Verlag, 2002: 1- 64.

Pui CH: Urate oxidase in the prophylaxis or treatment of hyperuricemia: the United States experience. Semin Hematol 2001; 38: 13–21.

Dyspnea and respiratory failure

12

M Bard
Erasmus Medical Centre, The Netherlands

Introduction

Dyspnea is commonly defined as an uncomfortable sensation or awareness of breathing. It is a particularly subjective sensation, with a complex pathophysiology in which both physical and cognitive factors play an important role. Dyspnea is generally reported to be frequent in the cancer population with prevalence variations related to the involvement of the cardiopulmonary system by the disease, the stage of cancer or the services (referral or palliative care) taking care of the patients. Cancer and its treatment are known precipitating factors for several diseases that involve the cardiopulmonary system, such as thromboembolic or infectious diseases. Moreover, cancer is commonly diagnosed in patients who have significant underlying cardiopulmonary problems, such as chronic obstructive pulmonary disease (COPD) or cardiac insufficiency.

Etiology

Etiologies of dyspnea are numerous in cancer patients and are more or less related to the cancer disease and/or its therapy. A non-exhaustive list of possible causes for dyspnea in the cancer patient is presented in Table 12.1.

Evaluation

Both history and physical examination are essential elements for the diagnosis and assessment of dyspnea. Medical, smoking and occupational histories and previous radiotherapy or chemotherapy provide important diagnostic information. The best source of information is the patient's self-report and the physical examination must rapidly evaluate the degree of respiratory failure and eliminate an extrathoracic cause.

Table 12.1 Causes of dyspnea

Relationship to cancer	Cause
Directly related to cancer	Primary/metastatic parenchymal lung involvement
	Airway obstruction
	Carcinomatous lymphangitis
	Pleural tumor
	Malignant pleural effusion
	Pericardial effusion
	Superior vena cava syndrome
	Tumor microemboli
	Phrenic nerve paralysis
	Atelectasis
	Tracheoesophageal fistula
	Chest wall invasion
	Pathological chest wall fracture
Indirectly related to cancer	Pneumonia
	Cachexia
	Electrolyte abnormalities
	Pulmonary embolus
	Paraneoplastic syndrome
	Ascites
Related to cancer therapy	Surgery (after lung or thorax wall resection)
	Radiation pneumonitis
	Chemotherapy-induced pulmonary fibrosis
	Chemotherapy-induced cardiomyopathy
Unrelated to cancer	Chronic obstructive pulmonary disease
	Asthma
	Interstitial lung disease
	Aspiration
	Pneumothorax
	Congestive heart failure
	Cardiac ischemia
	Arrhythmias
	Pulmonary vascular disease
	Obesity
	Neuromuscular disorders
	Anxiety

Anamnesis of the dyspnea

Quantitation

Patients describe dyspnea variously and sometimes use several misleading verbal expressions such as "fatigue" or "painful breathing." It is important to remember that the measurement of oxygen saturation is not correlated with dyspnea (patients may be hypoxemic but not dyspneic, or dyspneic but not hypoxemic). Functional assessment such as a walking test or the reading aloud of numbers have been validated but are rarely useful in an emergency context. Some evaluation scales such as the visual analog or the Borg scale can be used to simply and rapidly quantify dyspnea. Typically, these scales have a line with verbal descriptors (such as "no breathlessness" and "worst possible breathlessness" at the ends) on which the patient makes a mark that corresponds to the extent of the dyspnea.

History

The assessment of dyspnea should include a complete history of the symptom and should detail:

- The temporal onset – acute and chronic dyspnea are arbitrarily separated by an evolution of more or less than 2 weeks. Acute dyspnea is often less tolerated.
- The mode of occurrence – at rest or during exercise, nocturnal or diurnal.
- The presence of precipitating and relieving events or activities such as the position of the thorax (e.g. orthopnea), the cessation of an exercise or the intake of a medication (e.g. bronchodilator)
- The presence of associated symptoms such as thorax pain, fever, cough, sputum or hemoptysis.

Clinical examination

The clinical examination of the patient should detail:

- The respiratory frequency (in 1 minute) is a clinical parameter that should be systematically measured as the cardiac frequency and the peripheral blood pressure.
- The type of dyspnea (predominant during expiration or during inspiration). Inspiratory dyspnea suggests an upper airway obstruction (trachea, larynx) that is always an emergency. Expiratory dyspnea is common in bronchial disease such as asthma or COPD.

- The amplitude of the respiratory movement: deep and rapid, such as in metabolic acidosis (Kussmaul); cyclic with apneic period, such as in neurologic central disease (Cheyne–Stokes).
- The presence of thorax asymmetry or thorax deformation.
- The presence of added sounds such as stridor, rhonchi, sibilant or crepitations.
- The dullness of a hemithorax (pleural effusion, atelectasis).
- The presence of signs of cardiac insufficiency (left or right), vena cava syndrome, ascitis or peripheral phlebitis.

Complementary investigations

These investigations must be directed at the underlying cause and take into account their potential benefits for the patient. In an evident clinical context in a weak patient with an advanced disease, a simple clinical examination and a pulse oximetry measurement are sometimes sufficient to manage the symptom. It is important to remember that the measurements of arterial blood gas (PaO_2, $PaCO_2$) and pH values must be interpreted in relation to the patient's chronical status. In a general context, a first-line analysis of complementary investigations should associate:

- arterial blood gas with pH
- blood cell count with hemoglobin
- measurement of electrolytes with creatinine and liver function test
- glycemia
- electrocardiogram
- chest X-ray.

Evaluation of the tolerance

The research for signs of respiratory distress is rapidly completed. The presence of these signs induces a rapid management, with discussion of a transfer to an intensive care unit. Signs of bad tolerance are respiratory, hemodynamic and neuropsychic.

Respiratory

- Cyanosis, sweat.
- Polypnea or, conversely, bradypnea.
- Use of accessory respiratory muscles (intercostals, sternocleidomastoid).
- Paradoxal respiration (contraction of the abdominal muscles during inspiration, which is a sign of respiratory muscular exhaustion).

Hemodynamic
- Tachycardia.
- Hypotension, shock.

Neuropsychic
- Aggressiveness, agitation.
- Confusion, coma.

Elimination of an extrathoracic etiology

It is important to quickly diagnose these non-cardiopulmonary etiologies, which require specific managements.

Anemia (acute or chronic)
- Metabolic acidosis (diabetic ketoacidosis, renal failure, drug intoxication).
- Neurologic disorders (central or peripheral).

Management of dyspnea

The management of dyspnea must be adapted to the etiology and take into account the will of the patient and the stage of the cancer disease.

Oxygen

Oxygen is administered in case of hypoxemia without forgetting that hypoxemia and dyspnea are not correlated. The amount of administered oxygen is increased to reach an oxygen saturation level above 90–92%. For patients with chronic hypoventilation (such as patients suffering from COPD), the potential respiratory acidosis induction by high doses of oxygen must be controlled by an arterial blood gas (pH).

Corticosteroids

Corticosteroids can be used with various goals, such as the decrease of endobronchial inflammation in the case of acute asthma or COPD, the rapid improvement of a tumoral compression (vena cava syndrome, bronchial or vascular compression) or the improvement of a carcinomatous lymphangitis.

Bronchodilators

In the case of bronchospasm, bronchodilators (beta$_2$-agonist and anticholinergic) can be used. Nebulization is the first (and more efficient) way of administration for these drugs. Moreover, anticholinergic therapies have also been reported to decrease the secretion of sputum.

Opioids

In the case of patients with advanced cancer, the management concentrates on the symptoms and goals to relieve the patient's sense of the effort of breathing. Opioids have been reported to decrease exercise-induced dyspnea and to increase exercise tolerance in COPD or elderly patients. The mechanisms of action of opoids are not entirely clear but they can be safely and effectively used for the relief of dyspnea with a first administration at low dose (5 mg of morphine subcutaneously) and a careful titration during the first day of utilization.

Anxiolytics

The effectiveness of anxiolytic therapies on dyspnea relief has not been demonstrated. Theoretically, anxiolytics improve the dyspnea-related anxiety but, as for opioids, their utilization must be progressive and titrated in order to avoid a respiratory depression. In the case of refractory dyspnea, patient sedation can be discussed after informed consent.

Further reading

American Thoracic Society: Dyspnea, mechanisms, assessment, and management: a consensus statement. Am J Respir Crit Care Med 1999; 159: 321–40.

Ripamonti C, Fusco F: Respiratory problems in advanced cancer. Support Care Cancer 2002; 10: 204–16.

Thomas JR, von Gunten CF: Clinical management of dyspnea. Lancet Oncol 2002; 3: 223–8.

Pulmonary infections

B Besse
Hospital Germans Trias i Pujol, Spain

13

Introduction

There are four important steps to evaluate a patient with a pulmonary infection:

1. Information on symptoms and medical history (type of disease, evolution time of symptoms in time, risk factors such as anguillulosis or tuberculosis exposition, prophylactic treatment for infections, recent travel) should be collected.
2. The severity of the underlying immunodeficiency (neutropenic state, intensive chemotherapy, number of prior chemotherapy line(s), corticosteroid treatment, thoracic radiotherapy) should be evaluated.
3. A chest X-ray should be made
4. The severity of the acute event should be evaluated. This should lead to a decision regarding management as in- or outpatient, general medical ward or intensive care unit (ICU). This decision can be made with the pneumonia severity index (Table 13.1).

Evaluation

A summary of the evaluation is given in Table 13.2.

Eliminate a non-infectious disease

- Cancer: primary tumor, carcinomatous lymphangitis, pleural effusion, pulmonary leukostasis.
- Cardiac failure.
- Drug-induced lung disease: up-to-date information on www.pneumotox.com.
- Intra-alveolar hemorrhage.
- Pulmonary embolism.

Table 13.1 Pneumonia severity index (PSI)

Patient characteristic	Points assigned
Demographic factor	
Age:	
Male	Number of age
Female	Number of age − 10
Nursing home resident	+ 10
Comorbid illnesses:	
Active neoplastic disease	+ 30
Liver disease	+ 20
Congestive heart failure	+ 10
Cerebrovascular disease	+ 10
Renal disease	+ 10
Physical examination:	
Altered mental status	+ 20
Respiratory rate >30 breaths/minute	+ 20
Systolic blood pressure <90 mmHg	+ 20
Temperature <35°C or >40°C	+ 15
Pulse >125 beats/minute	+ 10
Laboratory or radiographic findings:	
Arterial pH >7.35	+ 30
Blood urea nitrogen >30 mg/dl	+ 20
Sodium <130 mEq/L	+ 10
Hematocrit <30%	+ 10
Arterial partial pressure of oxygen <60 mmHg	+ 10
Pleural effusion	+ 10

A total points score is obtained by adding the patient's age in years with the points for each applicable patient characteristic.

Interpretation of score:

   ≤90 total points: low risk

   91–130 points: moderate risk

   >130 points: high risk

Patients with 70< PSI scores ≤90 may require brief hospitalization.

Patients with PSI scores of greater than or equal to 91 total points are at significant increased risk for morbidity and mortality. These patients require hospitalization.

Table 13.2 Classical approach

Brutal beginning Fever Sepsis with ARDS	Rapid progression (a few days) Fever	Rapid to moderate progression (a few days to 1 month) Fever	Slow progression (more than 1 month) Absence or mild fever
Radiographic infiltrates	Diffuse opacities	Nodules or round infiltrates evolving towards dissemination and/or cavitation	Diffuse opacities
Bacterial pneumonia (*Streptococcus pneumoniae*, *Haemophilus influenzae*; to a lesser degree *Legionella* spp.)	Opportunistic pneumonia (pneumocystosis, cytomegalovirus, cryptococcosis, toxoplasmosis) Tuberculosis Hypersensitivity drug-induced pneumonitis	Fungal pneumonia ++ (bone marrow transplant) Legionellosis, tuberculosis, pulmonary embolus with pulmonary infarction or specific localization of vasculitis *Nocadia* sp.	Pulmonary edema Toxic treatment induces pneumonitis Non-specific pneumonitis (bone marrow transplant recipients)
Blood cultures ×2 Protected bronchial brushing in severe cases	Induced sputum (*Pneumocystis carinii*) Bronchoscopy with BAL	CT scan Bronchoscopy Lung biopsy if peripheral nodules	Echocardiography CT scan Bronchoscopy with BAL Lung biopsy if necessary

Pulmonary infections: etiology

The pathogens involved in pulmonary infections are given in Table 13.3.

Imaging and laboratory tests

Routine tests

- Complete blood cell and differential counts.
- Serum creatinine, urea nitrogen, glucose, electrolytes, bilirubin and liver enzyme values.
- O_2 saturation.

Table 13.3 Pathogens involved in pulmonary infections

Underlying immunodeficiencies or disease	Pathogens
Neutropenic patients <7 days of neutropenia	Gram-negative bacterial infections predominate, aerobic Gram-negative bacteria (Enterobacteriaceae, *Pseudomonas aeruginosa*), *Staphylococcus aureus*
Neutropenic patients: unfavorable course despite first-line antibiotics	*Staphylococcus* spp, nosocomial agents, and fungal infections (*Aspergillus*, *Zygomycetes*, *Fusarium* spp.) after 7 days of neutropenia
Impaired cellular immunity	Frequent: viral infections (cytomegalovirus, other herpesviruses), *Pneumocystis carinii* pneumonia More rarely bacterial (*Legionella*, *Nocardia*), mycobacterial, and fungal (*Aspergillus*, *Histoplasma*) infections
Impaired humoral immunity	Frequent: *Streptococcus pneumoniae* and *Haemophilus influenzae*
Primary or metastatic pulmonary neoplasms	Frequent: mixed bacterial etiology (*Staphylococcus* spp., Gram-negative bacilli, anaerobes) from postobstructive pneumonitis, lung abscess or empyema
Brain tumors and head and neck cancer	Organisms living in the oropharynx and upper airways in aspiration pneumonitis

■ Blood cultures (twice: once before treatment and once within the first 8 hours).
■ Gram stain and culture of sputum.

Indications for CT scan

■ Neutropenic patients: high-resolution computed tomograpy (CT) will reveal evidence of pneumonia in more than one-half of febrile neutropenic patients with normal findings on chest radiographs.

- Non-neutropenic patients:
  - respiratory symptoms or unexplained fever and a normal chest radiography
  - puzzling radiographic findings, initially or during the course of the condition
  - lung biopsy; CT scan is considered as guidance for the optimal type and site of biopsy.

Indications for bronchoscopy and bronchoalveolar lavage (BAL)

- Neutropenic patients: bronchoscopy and BAL can be safely done during aplastic period. BAL analysis is positive in about 57%. BAL should be done in the case of:
  - extensive pneumonia despite recommended empirical therapy
  - non-resolving pneumonia, even after the end of aplastic period
  - additional immune defect other than neutropenia and/or with unusual clinical presentation.
- Non-neutropenic patients: bronchoscopy with protected bronchial brushing (PBB) and BAL remains the cornerstone of definitive diagnosis of lung infection. Bronchoscopy with BAL is indicated as the first-line procedure in all cases except where there is a suspicion of embolism, edema or usual bacterial pneumonia. BAL results may be negative in case of aspergillosis, tuberculosis, nocardiosis or tumor.

In selected patients

- Test for *Legionella* in all seriously ill patients without an alternative diagnosis, especially if aged over 40 years old, immunocompromised or nonresponsive to beta-lactam antibiotics, if clinical features are suggestive of this diagnosis or in outbreak settings.
- Test for *Mycobacterium tuberculosis,* with acid-fast bacilli staining and culture in patients with a cough for several months, other common symptoms or suggestive radiographic changes.
- Outpatients: sputum Gram stain and culture for conventional bacteria are optional.

Treatment

Neutropenic patients

Neutropenic patients should be managed as in-patients. Empirical treatment with antibiotics should be started immediately (see Chapter 17).

Non-neutropenic patients

An attempt should be made to achieve pathogen-directed antimicrobial therapy (Table 13.4).

Empirical treatment for bacterial pneumonias

Patients with malignancies should be considered at risk of penicillin-resistant pneumococci. Intravenous (IV) treatment should be started immediately including:

- third-generation cephalosporin (cefotaxime 1 g every 8 hours or ceftriaxone 1 g every 24 hours) or
- combination of amoxicillin/clavulanate in case of lung cancer, head and neck cancer and brain tumors
- macrolide (erythromycin, total daily dose 2–4 g IV) should be added in order to treat legionnaires' disease; azithromycin or a fluoroquinolone can be used as well.

Duration of treatment

Duration of treatment is based on the pathogen, response to treatment, comorbidy and complications. The treatment should be at least as long as for immunocompetent patients:

- *Streptococcus pneumoniae*: 2 weeks
- *Staphylococcus aureus*, *Pseudomonas aeruginosa*, *Klebsiella*, anaerobes: at least 2 weeks (these bacteria can cause necrosis of pulmonary parenchyma)
- *Mycoplasma pneumoniae*, *Chlamydia pneumoniae*, legionnaires' disease: at least 2 weeks.

Route of administration

Intravenous therapy can be changed to oral therapy if the patient's condition is improving clinically and is hemodynamically stable; the patient is able to ingest the drug and the gastrointestinal tract is functioning normally (conditions met within 3 days in most cases). If no oral formulation of the IV drug is available, an oral agent with a similar spectrum of activity should be selected on the basis of in-vitro or predicted sensitivity patterns of the established or probable pathogen.

Table 13.4 Pathogen-directed antimicrobial therapy for community-acquired pneumonia

Organism	Preferred antimicrobial agent	Alternative microbial agent
Streptococcus pneumoniae		
Penicillin-susceptible	Penicillin G, amoxicillin	Cephalosporins, macrolides, fluoroquinolones
Penicillin-resistant	Fluoroquinolones, vancomycin	
Haemophilus influenzae	Cephalosporins (2nd–3rd generation), doxycycline, azithromycin	Fluoroquinolones, clarithromycin
Moraxella catarrhalis	Cephalosporins (2nd–3rd generation), macrolide	Fluoroquinolones
Anaerobes	®-lactam/®-lactamase inhibitor, clindamycin	Imipenem
Staphylococcus aureus		
Methicillin-susceptible	Nafcillin/oxacillin or gentamicin	Cefazolin or cefuroxime, vancomycin, clindamycin
Methicillin-resistant	Vancomycin or gentamicin	Linezolid
Enterobacteriaceae	Cephalosporin (3rd generation) ± aminoglycoside, carbapenem	Aztreonam, fluoroquinolone
Pseudomonas aeruginosa	Aminoglycoside + antipseudomonas β-lactam	Aminoglycoside + ciprofloxacin, ciprofloxacin + antipseudomonas β-lactam

Table 13.4 Continued

Organism	Preferred antimicrobial agent	Alternative microbial agent
Legionella	Macrolide + rifampicin, fluoroquinolone	Doxycycline + rifampicin
Mycoplasma pneumoniae	Doxycycline, macrolide	Fluoroquinolone
Chlamydia pneumoniae	Doxycycline, macrolide	Fluoroquinolone
Chlamydia psittaci	Doxycycline	Erythromycin
Nocardia	TMP-SMZ*	Imipenem + amikacin, doxycycline
Coxiella burnetrii	Tetracycline	Chloramphenicol
Influenzavirus	Amantadine or rimantadine (infl A), zanamivir (infl A+B)	–

*TMP-SMZ, trimethoprim–sulfamethoxazole.

Assessment of response to treatment

Objective parameters include:

- Pulmonary symptoms.
- Fever – time to defervescence is usually 2.5 days for pneumococcal pneumonia (until 6–7 days in bacteremic cases, or in elderly patients).
- Partial pressure of oxygen.
- Peripheral leukocyte count.
- Findings on serial radiographs – radiographic findings usually clear more slowly than clinical findings. Radiographic progression is possible during the first days of treatment, despite a good clinical response.
- Blood culture in case of bacteremic pneumonias: usually negative within 24 to 48 hours of treatment; *Pseudomonas aeruginosa* and *Mycoplasma pneumoniae* can persist despite effective therapy.

Failure to response

Different possibilities should be considered:

- Incorrect diagnosis.
- Host-related problems – obstruction by neoplasm, empyema, adverse drug reaction, pulmonary superinfection, sepsis from other causes (IV line).
- Drug-related problem – inappropriate dosing, problem of compliance, malabsorption, drug–drug interaction, drug reactions.
- Pathogen-related problems – resistant pathogen, non-identified pathogen.

Further reading

Bartlett JG, Dowell SF, Mandell LA et al: Practice guidelines for the management of community-acquired pneumonia in adults. Clin Infect Dis 2000; 31: 347–82.

Fine MJ, Auble TE, Yealy DM et al: A prediction rule to identify low-risk patients with community-acquired pneumonia. N Engl J Med 1997; 336: 243–50.

Kent A, Sepkowitz A: Opportunistic infections in patients with and patients without acquired immunodeficiency syndrome. Clin Infect Dis 2002; 34: 1098–107

Mayaud C, Cadranel J: A persistant challenge: the diagnosis of respiratory disease in the non-AIDS immunocompromised host. Thorax 2000; 55: 511–17.

Rolston KV: The spectrum of pulmonary infections in cancer patients. Curr Opin Oncol 2001; 14: 218–23.
www.pneumotox.com

Nausea and vomiting

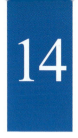

Y Mountzios
251 Air Force General Hospital, Greece

Introduction

Nausea and vomiting are two of the greatest fears of patients with cancer. They may be a result of the disease status of the patient but are more frequently associated with anti-cancer treatment. Inadequately controlled chemotherapy and radiation-induced nausea and vomiting can precipitate a number of medical complications that may prove life threatening, including dehydration and electrolyte imbalance, or cause physical damage, including Mallory–Weiss tears of the esophagus. The distressing symptoms of nausea and vomiting have a considerable impact on all aspects of the patients' quality of life, as well as those of their family and caregivers. The distress resulting from these symptoms can escalate over time and can potentially lead to a patient's refusal to continue with the most effective antitumor therapy.

Nausea and vomiting associated with chemotherapy can be classified as acute, delayed or anticipatory. Acute nausea and vomiting are defined as occurring within 24 hours after chemotherapy and can be further subdivided into acute (within 12 hours) and late-acute (12–24 hours). Delayed nausea and vomiting are usually defined as commencing more than 24 hours after administration of chemotherapy and may persist for 6–7 days. They commonly occur following the administration of cisplatin, carboplatin, cyclophosphamide or doxorubicin. Anticipatory nausea and vomiting occur before, during or after (but before acute chemotherapy symptoms would be expected to occur) the administration of a subsequent course of treatment if previous emetic control has been poor. They are conditioned responses linked to visual, gustatory, olfactory and environmental factors associated with previously administered chemotherapy.

Etiology

Nausea and vomiting have different etiologies.

Treatment-induced

- Chemotherapy: usually within the 5 days following the treatment (Table 14.1).
- Analgesics (e.g. opioids).
- Radiotherapy.

Metabolic causes

- Hypercalcemia.
- Renal failure.
- Adrenocortical failure.

Gastrointestinal causes

- Liver metastases or hepatitis.
- Biliary duct obstruction.
- Pancreatic disorders.
- Bowel obstruction (peritoneal carcinomatosis, colorectal cancer).
- Peritonitis.
- Gastric cancer.

Table 14.1 *Emetogenicity of chemotherapy*

Low emetogenic	Moderate emetogenic	Highly emetogenic
Bleomycin	Cyclophosphamide <750 mg/m^2	Carboplatin
Etoposide	Oral cyclophosphamide	Cisplatin
Gemcitabine	Ifosfamide	Carmustine
Methotrexate	Doxorubicin 20–60 mg/m^2	Cyclophosphamide
Fludarabine	Epirubicin <90 mg/m^2	>750 mg/m^2
Vinblastine	Idarubicin	Cytarabine
Vincristine	Oxaliplatin	>1000 mg/m^2
Vinorelbine	Irinotecan	Doxorubicin
Docetaxel	Methotrexate 250–1000 mg/m^2	>60 mg/m^2
Paclitaxel	Mitoxantrone <15 mg/m^2	Methotrexate
Mitomycin C		>1000 mg/m^2
		Dacarbazine
		Temozolomide
		Streptozotocin

Neurologic disorders

- Brain metastases with high intracranial pressure.
- Meningitis.

Other causes

- Myocardial infarction, renal failure.

Treatment

Check potential complications

Blood pressure, diuresis, creatininemia, kalemia, alkalosis, hematemesis.

Look for a cause if vomiting is not chemotherapy-related

Clinical examination

Abdomen/neurological examination/blood pressure/diuresis.

Blood examination

Liver tests, creatininemia, calcemia.

Technical examination

Ultrasonography, abdominal X-ray.

- If clinical examination suggests neurological disorder: brain computed tomography (CT) scan, lumbar puncture.
- If clinical examination suggests abdominal cause: abdominal CT scan.

Treatment of chemotherapy-related vomiting (prophylactic treatment excluded)

If moderate vomiting, without complication

- outpatient management, treatment with serotonin antagonist orally (or intrarectally) and/or metoclopramide and/or corticosteroids.
- check the evolution after 24 hours.

If severe or in case of complications

- hospitalization
- serotonin antagonist: e.g. granisetron: 3 mg × 1–2/day intravenously or ondansetron: 8 mg × 1–2/day intravenously and
- metoclopramide: 2 mg/kg/day intravenously and

- corticosteroids: prednisolone or methylprednisolone: 1–2 mg/kg/day intravenously
- in case of resistance: continuous intravenous perfusion of chlorpromazine 25 mg/day.

Further reading

ESMO Minimum Clinical Recommendations: Chemotherapy-induced nausea and vomiting. http://www.esmo.org/reference/reference_guidelines.htm

Gralla RJ: New agents, new treatment, and antiemetic therapy. Semin Oncol 2002; 29 (Suppl 4): 119–24.

Licitra L, Spinazze S, Roila F: Antiemetic therapy. Crit Rev Oncol Hematol 2002; 43: 93–101.

Mucositis

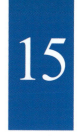

C Monnerat, N Ketterer
Centre Hospitalier Universitaire Vaudois, Suisse

Introduction

Oral mucositis is a significant problem in patients receiving chemotherapy or radiotherapy. Mucositis incidence is highly dependent on the treatment modalities. Among patients receiving standard chemotherapy, mucositis ranges from 10% to 40%, according to the type of chemotherapy. Virtually all patients who receive radiotherapy to the head and neck area develop oral complications. About 75% of the recipients of stem cell transplant have a significant oral mucositis.

Patients describe oropharyngeal mucositis as the most debilitating side effect. Mucositis is painful, may limit the nutritional intake and diminish the quality of life and thus decrease the patient's compliance. Severe mucositis with extensive ulceration often necessitates parenteral nutrition and use of narcotics, and may result in serious clinical complications, leading to prolonged hospitalizations. Finally, mucositis may result in the need to delay or reduce the dosage of subsequent chemotherapy or to delay radiotherapy, which ultimately may compromise the success of the therapy.

Pathophysiology

Normally, cells of the mouth undergo rapid renewal over a 7- to 14-day cycle. Both chemotherapy and radiotherapy interfere with cellular mitosis and reduce the regenerative ability of the oral mucosa. The mechanisms of the development and healing of mucositis have been described as a complex biologic process that occurs in four phases:

- An inflammatory or vascular phase, during which cytokines such as tumor necrosis factor-alpha (TNF-α) and interleukin-1 (IL-1) are released, damaging the epithelial cells and increasing the vascularity and the mucosal cytotoxic drug concentration.

- An epithelial phase with reduced epithelial renewal, causing mucosal atrophy and ulceration a few days after chemotherapy.
- An ulcerative or bacteriologic phase, where localized areas of erosion often become covered with a fibrinous pseudomembrane. As this phase usually coincides with the patient's period of maximum neutropenia, a rapid bacterial colonization occurs, stimulating further cytokine release.
- A healing phase, where there is a renewal of the mucosal epithelium, with normalization of the patient's peripheral white blood cell count and re-establishment of the local microbial flora.

Risk factors

The expected severity of the mucositis for an individual patient depends on the following factors.

Chemotherapy and radiotherapy

The type, dose and schedule of chemotherapy and the concomitant administration of radiotherapy are all factors that affect mucositis.

Patient's characteristics

- Young or older age has been associated with a more severe mucositis. Children experience severe mucositis, probably related to the higher rate of their mucosal renewal. Older patients receiving 5-fluorouracil (5-FU)-based chemotherapy tend to have a more frequent and severe mucositis.
- Female sex is an unexplained risk factor for 5-FU-induced mucositis. In a meta-analysis of 731 patients receiving 5-FU, the incidence of any mucositis for women was 63% versus 52% for men ($p = 0.002$) and the incidence of severe or very severe mucositis for women and men was 22% and 12%, respectively ($p = 0.0006$).
- Poor nutritional status associated with vitamin and protein/calorie deficiencies can interfere with mucosal regeneration by decreasing cellular renewal.
- Pre-existing mucosal damage caused by periodontal disease or ill-fitting dental prosthesis.
- Xerostomia before and during treatment is associated with a more severe mucositis.
- Smoking.
- Genetic susceptibilities for antimetabolites (methotrexate, 5-FU). Patients carrying the C677T polymorphism of the methylenetetrahydrofolate

reductase gene (MTHFR) have an increased susceptibility to methotrexate. Dihydropyrimidine dehydrogenase (DPD) deficiency is associated with an increased risk of toxicity in cancer patients receiving 5-FU treatment.

Evaluation

Scoring oral mucositis – the severity of the mucositis – can be assessed with several scales:

■ The World Health Organization (WHO) Mucositis Scale (Table 15.1) is the oldest score and measures accurately the clinical consequences of mucositis (i.e. pain and the requirement of parenteral medication and nutrition).
■ The National Cancer Institute Common Toxicity Criteria (NCI CTC) Mucositis Scale (Table 15.2) is mostly used in chemotherapy trials and is very similar to the WHO score. However, the WHO and the NCI CTC scores are too subjective to accurately represent the anatomic and pathophysiologic changes that occur during mucositis.

Table 15.1 World Health Organization Mucositis Scale

Grade	Description
Grade 0	None
Grade 1	Soreness/erythema
Grade 2	Erythema, ulcers, but able to eat solids
Grade 3	Ulcers; requires liquid diet
Grade 4	Oral alimentation not possible

Table 15.2 The National Cancer Institute Common Toxicity Criteria (NCI CTC) Mucositis Scale

Grade	Description
Grade 0	None
Grade 1	Painless ulcers, erythema or mild soreness
Grade 2	Painful erythema, edema, or ulcers; can eat
Grade 3	Painful erythema, edema, or ulcers; cannot eat
Grade 4	Requires parenteral or enteral support

- The Radiation Therapy Oncology Group (RTOG) Mucositis Scale (Table 15.3) describes more precisely the appearance of the mouth lesions, but without anatomic considerations.
- The Oral Mucositis Assessment Scale (OMAS) (Table 15.4) is a strictly observational tool that measures lesion size and erythema at nine different sites in the oral cavity. This very precise scale is particularly useful for the assessment of the mucositis experienced by head and neck cancer patients. However, this scale needs an experienced observer and is difficult to use in patients with severe pain.

Table 15.3 The Radiation Therapy Oncology Group (RTOG) Mucositis Scale

Grade	Description
Grade 0	No change over baseline
Grade 1	Injection; may experience mild pain not requiring analgesic
Grade 2	Patchy mucositis, may have a serosanguinuous discharge; may experience pain requiring analgesics
Grade 3	Confluent fibrinous mucositis; may include severe pain requiring narcotics
Grade 4	Ulceration, hemorrhage or necrosis

Table 15.4 Oral Mucositis Assessment Scale (OMAS)

Location	Ulceration/pseudomembrane*	A Erythema[†]
Upper lip	0, 1, 2, 3	0, 1, 2
Lower lip	0, 1, 2, 3	0, 1, 2
Right cheek	0, 1, 2, 3	0, 1, 2
Left cheek	0, 1, 2, 3	0, 1, 2
Right vertical/lateral tongue	0, 1, 2, 3	0, 1, 2
Left vertical/lateral tongue	0, 1, 2, 3	0, 1, 2
Floor of mouth	0, 1, 2, 3	0, 1, 2
Soft palate	0, 1, 2, 3	0, 1, 2
Hard palate	0, 1, 2, 3	0, 1, 2

*0 = none; 1 = <1 cm^2; 2 = 1–3 cm^2; 3 = >3 cm^2.
[†]0 = none; 1 = not severe; 2 = severe.

The use of these different scales has made difficult the comparison between studies and there is currently not a universally accepted scale.

Prevention and treatment of mucositis

Many therapeutic interventions have been tried in the management of mucositis, but few randomized clinical trials have been performed to establish strong clinical guidelines. Most trials have included too few patients and have not had sufficient statistical power to conclude on the efficacy of the preventive measure under study. The use of various scoring systems and different clinical endpoints has made a comparison between trials hazardous and completion of meta-analysis difficult.

Oral hygiene

Effective prevention of mucositis requires the correction of poor oral hygiene and the treatment of any dental diseases that could be a potential source of infection. Oral hygiene programs are commonly advised to reduce the amount and activity of oral microflora and to prevent or reduce discomfort associated with oral mucositis. However, the superiority of an intensive oral hygiene protocol involving initial treatment of dental lesions and tooth and gum brushing during bone marrow aplasia was not clinically useful compared to a limited oral hygiene protocol in bone marrow transplantation patients. In the same clinical setting, an older trial found that maintenance of good oral hygiene was beneficial.

As a general rule, every cancer patient should be instructed to keep an adequate oral hygiene to minimize the risk of mucositis. Soft toothbrushes should be used in a non-traumatic way with fluoridated toothpaste. Once mucosal damage has occurred, rinsing solution only should be preferred. Moisture of the oral mucosa should be maintained by sufficient hydration. Use of sugarless chewing gum can stimulate salivary production. Lipstick lubricants can be applied frequently.

Mouthwashes

In order to keep an adequate oral mucosa moisture and hygiene, frequent mouthwashes are recommended. Several mouthrinses, including simple saline rinses, bicarbonate rinses and chlorhexidine rinses, are available. Alcohol-containing rinses are too irritant and should be avoided. A trial comparing three different mouthwashes – a saline and bicarbonate rinse, a chlorhexidine-containing rinse and a lidocaine (lignocaine) and antacid (such as magnesium)-

containing rinse – demonstrated the same efficacy on the duration of mucositis and intensity of symptoms.

Trials evaluating prostaglandin, glutamine, granulocyte–macrophage colony-stimulating factor or GM-CSF (molgramostim), chamomile and allopurinol mouthrinses were judged as not conclusive in a meta-analysis.

Oral cooling

Oral cooling (cryotherapy) probably causes local vasoconstriction and, thus, temporarily reduces oral mucosal blood flow and the amount of the drug delivered to oral mucosa cells. Patients are taught to swish ice chips in their mouths for a total of 30 minutes, starting 5 minutes prior to each dose of chemotherapy. Ice chips were shown to be effective in the meta-analysis (relative risk 0.57; 95% CI 0.43–0.77). Four patients needed to be treated to prevent one extra case of mucositis over the baseline incidence. Oral cooling using ice cubes during a 5-FU infusion could halve the incidence of 5FU-induced stomatitis.

Sucralfate

Sucralfate is a basic aluminum salt whose action may involve its binding to the damaged mucosal surface proteins and the formation of a protective coating over the ulcer. Results of 14 trials are controversial and the use of sucralfate is dependent on the institution's experience. A recent trial showed that sucralfate mouthwash for prevention and treatment of 5FU-induced mucositis was not better than the usual prevention with ice cubes. In another small randomized study in 30 head and neck patients receiving chemoradiotherapy, addition of sucralfate to a mouthwash was of no benefit.

Antimicrobial agents

In neutropenic patients, an intact mucosa is an important host defense against systemic bacterial and fungal infections, including viridans streptococcus, enterococcus, anaerobic bacteria and certain Gram-negative bacteria. Between 25% and 50% of cases of septicemia in neutropenic cancer patients appear to originate from oral colonizing bacteria. It has been estimated that, when a patient under chemotherapy dies from an infection, the causative organism originates in the oral cavity for half of the cases. As a severe mucositis is an important contributory factor to a systemic infection in neutropenic patients, the reduction of bacterial, fungal or viral colonization of the oropharynx could reduce the rate of secondary infections associated with mucositis and reduce its severity. Several topical antimicrobials have been studied as prophylactic agents:

- Use of chlorhexidine rinses was not beneficial.
- Polymyxin B, tobramycin and amphotericin B (PTA) containing lozenges have shown a small clinical benefit in two randomized studies in head and neck cancer patients receiving radiotherapy, but a recent larger trial found that a PTA paste did not reduce the incidence of mucositis.
- In a meta-analysis of 15 studies, there was evidence that antifungal agents that are partially or fully absorbed from the gastrointestinal tract prevent oral candidiasis and that the partially absorbed agents (such as nystatin or amphotericin B) may be more effective than the fully absorbed agents. In patients with a long-duration neutropenia, nystatin or amphotericin B mouthwash are frequently prescribed, although strong evidence of their efficacy remains controversial.

Acyclovir

The risk for reactivation of a herpes simplex virus (HSV) correlates with the dose intensity of antineoplastic therapy. Reactivation occurs in up to 70–80% of seropositive bone marrow transplant (BMT) and acute leukemic patients. It should be noted that a chemotherapy-induced mucositis is difficult to differentiate clinically from a viral mucositis.

Acyclovir prophylaxis has been shown to be effective in preventing oropharyngeal shedding of the virus in HSV-seropositive patients receiving intensive chemotherapy for acute leukemia with a decrease in the number of nonfungal oral infections and also in patients undergoing stem cell transplantation.

Two nonrandomized studies have recently shown that oral valacyclovir appears as effective as intravenous acyclovir in preventing reactivation of HSV infection in autologous stem cell recipients.

Acyclovir or valacyclovir prophylaxis may thus be recommended for HSV-seropositive patients receiving autologous stem cell transplantation or other high-dose chemotherapy.

Protection of epithelial cells

Drugs that protect the normal tissue while maintaining the tumoricidal action of radiotherapy would be effective in the prevention of mucositis. Amifostine is a phosphorylated aminothiol prodrug that scavenges the free radicals created by the radiation. A large randomized trial in head and neck cancer patients has shown a decrease rate of xerostomia, but no change in the rate of grade 3 mucositis.

Enhancement of the epithelial proliferation would accelerate the healing phase of mucositis. GM-CSF could influence the proliferation of keratinocytes. However, clinical efficacy of the systemic as well as the local application of GM-CSF could not be confirmed and the cost of this treatment was prohibitive.

General supportive care
Pain management
Pain is a common complication of mucositis that could compromise an adequate oral hydration and nutrition of the patient. Topical anesthetics such as a lidocaine (lignocaine)-containing mixture can produce temporary pain relief to allow swallowing. Topical morphine for mucositis-associated pain following concomitant chemoradiotherapy for head and neck carcinoma was shown to reduce the need for systemic opiates and the duration of pain associated with the mucositis was shortened. However, patients with severe discomfort may need narcotics for their pain management. Sustained-release oral doses, transdermal application or continuous intravenous infusion of morphine or derivates may be required.

Nutritional support
Chemoradiotherapy for patients with squamous cell head and neck carcinoma is associated with mucositis and dysphagia that is so severe that enteral nutritional support becomes mandatory. Patient preference has resulted in the increasing use of percutaneous endoscopic gastrostomy (PEG) tubes rather than nasogastric (NG) tubes. It is possible that a PEG tube is required for a longer period of time and is associated with more persistent dysphagia. It is not known if a better nutritional support can lessen the severity and duration of the mucositis, but the comfort of the patient is dramatically improved.

Conclusion
The prevention and management of oral mucositis remains unsatisfactory, and the existing approaches amount to little more than common sense. The Oncology Nursing Society has recently published guidelines for the management of mucositis in head and neck cancer patients (Table 15.5). These guidelines can be adopted for the management of uncomplicated mucositis in any cancer patient, but additional measures can be applied, such as the use of pre-

Table 15.5 *Minimal clinical practice guidelines for mucositis*

Guideline	Description
1	Dental consult prior to initiation of cancer treatment for patients with head and neck malignancies or acute leukemia
2	Patient education prior to treatment initiation
3	At least three times daily oral assessment by the patient or the nurse and application of the following measures:
3a	Brush teeth with soft toothbrush and fluoride toothpaste (brushing is contraindicated in individuals with low platelets or gingival hemorrhage)
3b	Mouth rinses with normal saline or sodium bicarbonate Alcoholic mouthwash or chlorhexidine mouthwash are not recommended for mucositis prevention
3c	Topical fluoride for dental hygiene and caries prevention
3d	Mouth moisturizer to lips and oral cavity
4	Topical analgesic such as lidocaine (lignocaine) (avoid various compounded formulations)

ventive mouth cooling or the addition of nystatin-containing mouthwashes for neutropenic patients. Mucositis remains an important clinical issue in the daily management of cancer patients: consequences on the quality of life of the patients and on the therapy outcomes are underestimated. Further larger studies are still warranted in this field.

Further reading

Barasch A, Peterson DE: Risk factors for ulcerative oral mucositis in cancer patients: unanswered questions. Oral Oncol 2003; 39: 91–100.

Common Toxicity Criteria, Version 2.0, 1999.

Cox JD, Stetz J, Pajak TF: Toxicity criteria of the Radiation Therapy Oncology Group (RTOG) and the European Organization for Research and Treatment of Cancer (EORTC). Int J Radiat Oncol Biol Phys 1995; 31: 1341–6.

Dodd MJ, Dibble SL, Miaskowski C et al: Randomized clinical trial of the effectiveness of 3 commonly used mouthwashes to treat chemotherapy-induced mucositis. Oral Surg Oral Med Oral Pathol Oral Radiol Endo 2000; 90: 39–47.

Mead GM: Management of oral mucositis associated with cancer chemotherapy. Lancet 2002; 359: 815–16.

Parulekar W, Mackenzie R, Bjarnason G, Jordan RC: Scoring oral mucositis Oral Oncol 1998; 34: 63–71.

Plevova P: Prevention and treatment of chemotherapy- and radiotherapy induced oral mucositis: a review. Oral Oncol 1999; 34: 453–70.

Relling MV, Dervieux T: Pharmacogenetics and cancer therapy. Nat Rev Cancer 2001; 1: 99–108.

Rogers BB: Mucositis in the oncology patient. Nurs Clin North Am 2001; 36 745–60.

Schubert MM: Oropharyngeal mucositis. Cambridge: Cambridge University Press, 1998.

Sonis ST, Fey EG: Oral complications of cancer therapy. Oncology (Huntingt 2002; 6: 680–6.

Sonis ST, Eilers JP, Epstein JB et al: Validation of a new scoring system fo the assessment of clinical trial research of oral mucositis induced by radia tion or chemotherapy. mucositis Study Group. Cancer 1999; 85: 2103–13.

Stricker CT, Sullivan J: Evidence-based oncology oral care clinical practice guidelines: development, implementation, and evaluation. Clin J Onco Nurs 2003; 7: 222–7.

Trotti A, Bellm LA, Epstein JB et al: Mucositis incidence, severity and associ ated outcomes in patients with head and neck cancer receiving radiothera py with or without chemotherapy: a systematic literature review. Radiothe Oncol 2003; 66: 253–62.

World Health Organization: Handbook for reporting results of cance treatment. Geneva: World Health Organization, 1979.

Worthington HV, Clarkson JE: Prevention of oral mucositis and oral candidia sis for patients with cancer treated with chemotherapy. Cochran systematic Review. J Dent Educ 2002; 66: 903–11.

Anemia in cancer

K Strasser-Weippl, H Ludwig
Wilhelminenspital, Austria

Introduction

Anemia is defined as a reduced number of circulating erythrocytes in peripheral blood or as a reduced level of hemoglobin (Hb). Anemia can be graded by considering the hemoglobin as mild, moderate, severe and life-threatening. The criteria of the World Health Organization and of the National Cancer Institute grading anemia according to Hb are given in Table 16.1.

Anemia can be found in over 30% of cancer patients. Its incidence increases with ongoing treatment and disease progression and depends on several conditions such as age, tumor type, histology and stage of the tumor, the presence or absence of infections and other co-morbidities.

Tumor types associated with an increased risk of anemia include lymphomas, multiple myeloma, gynecologic and genitourinary tumors and lung cancer. In general, the prevalence of anemia is lower in patients with solid tumors, although mild to moderate anemia is still very frequent.

In a recent survey that investigated the prevalence of anemia in 15 367 European cancer patients (European Cancer Anaemia Survey, ECAS), anemia defined by a Hb level <12 g/dl was present in 39% of patients. The highest

Table 16.1 *Grading of anemia according to the World Health Organization (WHO) and the National Cancer Institute (NCI)*

Severity	WHO	NCI
Grade 0 (within normal limits)	>11.0 g/dl	Within normal limits
Grade 1 (mild)	9.5–10.9 g/dl	10.0 g/dl to normal limits
Grade 2 (moderate)	8.0–9.4 g/dl	8.0–9.9 g/dl
Grade 3 (serious/severe)	6.5–7.9 g/dl	6.5–7.9 g/dl
Grade 4 (life-threatening)	<6.5 g/dl	<6.5 g/dl

prevalence of anemia was found in patients with persistent or recurrent disease (48%), whereas newly diagnosed patients and those in remission were less likely to be anemic (35% and 31%, respectively). Patients with hematologic malignancies and those receiving chemotherapy were especially prone to anemia (53% and 50%, respectively).

Etiology

Box 16.1 shows causes of anemia.

Chronic anemia of cancer

Anemia in patients with cancer is usually due to the underlying malignancy and/or due to cancer therapy, but all other types of anemia may occur in cancer patients as well. The most common cause of anemia in cancer is the so-called anemia of chronic disease (ACD), characterized by a normocytic, normochromic and hyporegenerative anemia with decreased serum iron and transferrin saturation (<20%), with normal or increased ferritin levels. It is caused by inflammatory cytokines – interleukin 1 (IL-1), tumor necrosis fac-

Box 16.1 Causes of anemia

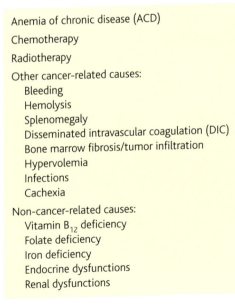

Anemia of chronic disease (ACD)

Chemotherapy

Radiotherapy

Other cancer-related causes:
  Bleeding
  Hemolysis
  Splenomegaly
  Disseminated intravascular coagulation (DIC)
  Bone marrow fibrosis/tumor infiltration
  Hypervolemia
  Infections
  Cachexia

Non-cancer-related causes:
  Vitamin B_{12} deficiency
  Folate deficiency
  Iron deficiency
  Endocrine dysfunctions
  Renal dysfunctions

tor (TNF) and interferon gamma (INF-gamma) – induced by the tumor, which lead to reduced erythropoietin (EPO) production, a decreased response of erythroid precursors to EPO and impaired iron utilization. Furthermore, the life span of erythrocytes is reduced.

Chemotherapy- and/or radiotherapy-induced anemia

Chemotherapy with myelosuppressive agents usually leads to transient anemia but increasing, cumulative doses of cytotoxic agents may eventually result in permanent erythropoietic insufficiency with irreversible, severe anemia. In addition, the renal toxic effects of certain chemotherapeutic agents can result in a blunted EPO response. Localized radiotherapy is often associated with only mild anemia or even without impairment of erythropoiesis, but radiotherapy to extended fields often causes anemia or aggravates pre-existing anemia.

Other causes of anemia in cancer

Apart from ACD, complications of cancer such as bleeding, hemolysis, splenomegaly, disseminated intravascular coagulation (DIC), bone marrow fibrosis or tumor infiltration, hypervolemia, infections and cachexia can lead to anemia in patients with cancer.

Other causes of anemia

Anemia in cancer may also be caused by factors not directly related to the disease or its treatment. Among these, vitamin B_{12} deficiency, folate and iron deficiency, as well as endocrine and renal dysfunctions are most frequent.

Evaluation

Anemia can cause symptoms and signs in many organ systems:

- Severe anemia leads to a release of vasoactive substances, which in turn lead to vasodilatation and reduced peripheral vessel resistance. Cardiac hyperactivity is the main compensatory mechanism in anemia and is felt by the patient as palpitations and pounding pulse (Table 16.2). In severe anemia, cardiac decompensation and congestive heart failure may evolve. The typical cardiovascular symptoms of anemia comprise fatigue, shortness of breath and palpitations, particularly during and following exercise.
- An increase in the respiratory rate in order to elevate blood oxygenation is a further important compensatory mechanism in anemia. Dyspnea, the corresponding symptom perceived by the patient, usually worsens if pulmonary edema occurs as a consequence of congestive heart failure.

Table 16.2 Organs affected by anemia and symptoms felt by the patient

Organ	Symptom
Heart	Palpitations, pounding pulse
Lung	Dyspnea
Kidney	Edema
Gastrointestinal	Nausea, anorexia
Skin	Pallor, reduced skin elasticity, broken nails
Immune system	Infections
Brain	Vertigo, dizziness, tinnitus, headache
Genitourinary	Loss of libido, impotence

■ In mild to moderate anemia, renal function is not impaired, but renal perfusion decreases with increasing anemia. This may result in fluid retention, hypervolemia, edema and cardiac decompensation.

■ Disturbances of the gastrointestinal tract do occur quite frequently in anemic patients but are often not recognized as a consequence of anemia. The underlying mechanism is a blood shift from the mesenteric and iliac beds to other areas of the body such as the central nervous system (CNS). Clinically, nausea and anorexia and, in advanced anemia, malabsorption may ensue.
A cardinal symptom of anemia is the pallor of mucous membranes, particularly of the mouth and pharynx, the conjunctivae, the lips and nail beds. Other changes of the skin include pale palms, reduced skin elasticity and broken nails.

■ Studies in patients on dialysis and in patients with iron deficiency revealed a negative impact of anemia on immune function, possibly through reduced secretion of Il-2 by peripheral blood mononuclear cells. In addition, the decreased perfusion of mucous membranes may facilitate infections, which may in turn aggravate anemia.

■ Impaired cerebral perfusion may lead to neurologic symptoms such as vertigo, dizziness, tinnitus and headache. The relationship of cognitive function with the degree of anemia has been documented in several studies.

■ Genitourinary symptoms may reach from menorrhagia, irregular menstrual cycles and amenorrhea, mainly caused by an impaired secretion of sexual hormones, to the loss of libido, and impotence in men.

■ Impact on quality of life (QoL): the impairment of organ function by anemia results in decreased QoL, with fatigue, depression, insomnia and reduced cognitive function as frequent symptoms. Many patients adapt to these dismal circumstances and often do not report diminished well-being. These patients are often surprised about the magnitude of subjective improvement when Hb levels are corrected by adequate therapy.

■ Impact on prognosis and on tumor biology: anemia is a negative prognostic factor in almost all types of cancer. Due to its predictive importance, Hb has been included as a predictive parameter in the Durie–Salmon staging system for myeloma and in the Binet staging system for chronic lymphocytic leukemia (CLL). Anemia correlates with tumor hypoxia, which induces a key regulator gene, hypoxia-inducible factor-1α (HIF-<). This regulatory gene induces transcription of a variety of genes important in angiogenesis, cell proliferation, drug and radiotherapy resistance. The consequence of this cascade is a more malignant tumor phenotype, leading to enhanced tumor growth, reduced sensitivity to tumor therapy and finally to reduced survival.

Treatment

Blood transfusions

Before the introduction of recombinant human erythropoietin, red blood cell (RBC) transfusions were the only effective therapy in anemic patients. One package of RBCs contains approximately 1.7×10^{12} erythrocytes in a volume of 270 ml. This is equivalent to an Hb value of 24 g/dl and a hematocrit level of 70%. The administration of RBC transfusions leads to a rapid increase in Hb level and improvement of anemia.

Indications

RBC transfusions are usually only indicated in severely anemic and symptomatic patients and are recommended at Hb levels ≤8 g/dl. RBC transfusions lead to an increase in Hb in almost all patients but the effect is transient and lasts only about 2 weeks. Importantly, the impact on QoL is usually small or modest, because the common target Hb level (10 g/dl) for treatment with RBC corresponds to the trigger point for initiation of erythropoietin therapy. Even when higher trigger points are chosen, the improvement in anemia-related QoL often remains inadequate.

Limitations

Due to the transient improvement in Hb, further transfusions will be required after a few weeks. This leads to quite varying Hb levels with repeating phases of decreased QoL and increased symptoms of anemia. In addition, fluctuating Hb levels may impair the physiological compensatory mechanisms to anemia, e.g. an increase in cardiac output. Although several studies have tried to identify predictive factors for the future need of transfusions, Hb level is still the only factor significantly associated with a repeated need of RBC.

Transfusions lead to febrile reactions in up to 10% of patients, sometimes accompanied by chills, headache and malaise. They are usually due to sensitization to HLA leukocyte and plasma antigens and due to contamination of the RBCs with bacterial antigens and pyrogens. ABO and Rh-incompatibility are rare and usually the result of human mistake, but they may be severe to life-threatening. A further important risk is the transfer of infections, although advances in testing for contaminating viruses and preparation of RBCs have made transfusions relatively safe.

Repeated transfusions bear the risk of iron overload, as with each RBC package 200–250 mg of iron are transfused. The resulting hemochromatosis may lead to liver damage and impaired heart capacity through accumulation of iron in the myocardium. Several studies indicate that RBCs are immunosuppressive and may impair outcome in transfused patients. Graft-versus-host disease is rare and predominantly seen in patients with hematologic malignancies. The production of antibodies against red cell antigens leads to alloimmunization and a reduced effectiveness of RBC transfusions.

The result is an increased need for transfusions after shorter intervals, which is further enhanced by suppression of endogenous erythropoietin production. With patients becoming increasingly aware of these risks, they may be reluctant to take RBC transfusions until their symptoms from anemia have become very severe.

Apart from these medical risks, there are logistical and financial considerations arguing against the routine use of RBC transfusions. As transfusions have to be given in a hospital environment, the cost of administration is high and patient autonomy is reduced. The cost per package is further raised by more stringent selection of potential donors and increasingly vigorous testing of transfusions. In 2003, the total cost of a single allogeneic RBC package in the United States was $550. Considering the facts discussed above, reservation is called for when prescribing RBC transfusions for the treatment of anemia.

Advantages

There are clear indications for the use of transfusions in anemic patients. First, RBC transfusions are the only treatment delivering a fast relief of symptoms in severely anemic patients. If a patient suffers from dyspnea or fatigue, the administration of transfusions prior to the start of erythropoietin treatment should be considered. Furthermore, treatment with erythropoietic agents is ineffective in about 30–40% of tumor patients. In these patients RBC transfusions should be used for the correction of anemia.

Erythropoietic agents

Erythropoietin (EPO) is an endogenous hormone produced by the kidneys, which, by binding to the erythropoietin receptor on erythroid colony-forming units, regulates erythropoiesis. Eryhthropoietin production is stimulated by tissue hypoxia. Since 1985, recombinant human erythropoietin has been available for use in anemic patients. The first erythropoietin introduced into the clinic was erythropoietin-alpha with erythropoietin-beta following a few years later. Both erythropoietins share the same amino acid structure. The glycosylation of erythropoietin-alpha is nearly identical to native erythropoietin, whereas erythropoietin-beta has less sialic acids. Numerous studies were conducted in patients with hematological malignancies and solid tumors, showing the effectiveness of both erythropoietins in improving Hb levels and symptoms of anemia and decreasing the need for RBC transfusions. It was also demonstrated that many anemic cancer patients suffer from erythropoietin deficiency when compared to patients with other types of anemia.

Darbepoietin-alpha, a novel erythropoiesis stimulating protein (NESP), was developed recently and is currently being evaluated in clinical trials for the treatment and prevention of anemia in cancer patients. It has a longer serum half-life than erythropoietin but a lower receptor affinity.

CERA (continuous erythropoiesis receptor activator) is another new erythropoietic drug with a prolonged serum half-life, which is currently in phase II studies in cancer patients.

Many cancer patients, even those not initially anemic, develop anemia during the further course of their disease. This is particularly true for patients receiving chemotherapy and especially for those being treated with platinum-containing regimens. Although young, physically fit patients may tolerate mild to moderate anemia quite well, middle-aged and elderly patients and those with co-morbidities may suffer from symptoms even at minor reductions of Hb levels. Hence, prevention of anemia should be considered in patients at risk for impairment of QoL due to a decrease in Hb levels. Indeed, several studies have now confirmed the potential of erythropoietins to prevent the development of anemia and the anemia-associated decline in QoL in patients subjected to chemotherapy. As this issue is presently still evolving, consensus guidelines on the use of erythropoietic agents for prevention have as yet not been established.

Indications

Present ASCO/ASH guidelines recommend initiation of erythropoietin treatment at a Hb level of ≤10 g/dl (Box 16.2). Treatment should also be considered at higher Hb levels (≤12 g/dl) if the patient suffers from symptoms of anemia. The largest benefit from treatment can be expected when the Hb level is boosted from 10 to 12 g/dl. A more patient-centered approach argues for the treatment of anemia in any patient suffering from anemia-related symptoms and/or an impairment of QoL. Following this approach, young, otherwise healthy individuals with slowly evolving anemia may not need treatment even in the presence of severe anemia, whereas multimorbid, elderly persons with early development of symptoms may need correction of anemia even at higher Hb levels than mentioned in the guidelines.

The standard dose of 10 000 IU thrice or 30 000–40 000 IU weekly should be customized to a target Hb value of 12 g/dl. This means that if no response is noted after 4 weeks, the dose should be increased to 20 000 IU thrice or

Box 16.2 *Treatment guidelines for erythropoietic agents*

Treatment indications

Hb ≤10 g/dl

or

Hb ≤12 g/dl and symptoms of anemia

Dosing of erythropoietin

Start:	10 000 × 3/week or 30 000–40 000/week → target Hb = 12 g/dl
No response:	20 000 × 3/week or 60 000/week → stop if not successful

Dosing of darbepoietin*

Start:	2.25 µg/kg once weekly → target Hb = 12 g/dl
No response:	increase dose by 50% → stop if not successful
Hb increase beyond 14 g/dl:	stop and restart when Hb <12 g/dl

*Based on expert recommendations

60 000 IU weekly, and if there is still no response at these dose levels, therapy with EPO should be discontinued. This is also the case if an Hb level of >14 g/dl is reached, but in these patients EPO treatment should be restarted at a lower dose if the Hb level falls below 12 g/dL again.

The recommended dose for darbepoietin is 2.25 µg/kg/week. Several trials have shown that longer treatment intervals up to 3 weeks may be feasible with higher darbepoietin doses. In case of no or insufficient response in the initial treatment phase, dose increments of 50% should be used, similarly to EPO.

Overall, 50–70% of cancer patients will respond to EPO treatment. The median time to response is approximately 4 weeks, but, including a possible dose increase, it can take up to 12 weeks to determine responsiveness. Factors predicting a good response include stable disease, low endogenous levels of erythropoietin (<100 mU/ml) and adequate bone marrow function. The likelihood of response is decreased in the presence of additional complications such as infections, in the case of functional iron deficiency, if the patient is undergoing concomitant aggressive anticancer treatment or if there is a history of excessive need for RBC transfusions.

Limitations

The most important disadvantages of erythropoietin compared to RBC transfusions are the long time interval until the Hb level is improved and the fact that not all patients respond to treatment. Other risks include aggravation of pre-existing hypertension, particularly in patients with chronic renal failure, and a worsening of splenomegaly in patients with myeloproliferative disorders. Furthermore, treatment with EPO leads to an increased risk of developing thromboembolic events (relative risk 1.55), particularly in persons with a previous history of thromboembolic complications. In selected patients, treatment with low molecular weight heparin or oral anticoagulants might be indicated. A rare, but severe complication in EPO-treated patients on chronic hemodialysis is pure red cell aplasia, which seems to be prevented simply by storing the drug correctly (at 4–6°C). The discussion about whether recombinant human erythropoietin is able to stimulate tumor growth was driven by in-vitro studies with inconclusive results. Further investigations are clearly warranted regarding this issue. Finally, the cost of treatment with erythropoietin is prohibitively high in many countries and limits its widespread use, even in the developed world.

Advantages

The major advantage of the use of erythropoietin for treating anemia is obviously that the numerous risks and downsides of administering RBC transfusions can be avoided. Although the need for transfusions can be totally abrogated in only 1 out of 3–4 patients treated with EPO, the Hb level is increased in 50–70% of patients. Furthermore, the association of EPO use with improved QoL and functional capacity independent of tumor response has been well established in clinical studies. In breast cancer patients undergoing adjuvant treatment, EPO was even shown to prevent the decline in cognitive function associated with chemotherapy.

Iron supplementation

All patients suffering from iron deficiency (transferrin saturation <20%) should be offered iron supplementation. In anemic patients treated with erythropoietic agents, functional iron deficiency is a major predictive factor. Therefore, ferritin levels should be kept above 300 µg/L and transferrin saturation above 20% during therapy. Although the results from a recently published study suggest that parenteral iron supplementation is more effective than oral administration, long-term intravenous iron replacement cannot be recommended because of possible immunosuppression and tumor growth promotion.

Conclusion

Anemia is a common condition in cancer patients. Its consequences reach from a reduced quality of life in patients with otherwise no symptoms of anemia, to life-threatening complications such as heart failure and cachexia. Furthermore, anemia may lead to a decreased tumor response to radio- or chemotherapy. Correcting and preventing anemia is therefore of paramount importance in cancer patients. Although this can easily be achieved by administering blood transfusions, they are associated with several side effects and risks and their impact on Hb level is transient. In 50–70% of cancer patients, anemia can be treated more effectively with erythropoietic agents (erythropoietin and darbepoietin). In most patients, treatment with erythropoietic agents leads to a stable improvement in Hb levels, quality of life and functional capacity.

Further reading

Barrett-Lee PJ, Bailey NP, O'Brien ME, Wager E: Large-scale UK audit of blood transfusion requirements and anaemia in patients receiving cytotoxic chemotherapy. Br J Cancer 2000; 82: 93–7.

Faulds D, Sorkin EM: Epoetin (recombinant human erythropoietin). A review of its pharmacodynamic and pharmacokinetic properties and therapeutic potential in anaemia and the stimulation of erythropoiesis. Drugs 1989; 38: 863–99.

Gordon MS: Managing anemia in the cancer patient: old problems, future solutions. Oncologist 2002; 7: 331–41.

Koeller JM: Clinical guidelines for the treatment of cancer-related anemia. Pharmacotherapy 1998; 18: 156–69.

Ludwig H, Fritz E: Anemia in cancer patients. Semin Oncol 1998; 25: 2–6.

Ludwig H, Strasser K: Symptomatology of anemia. Semin Oncol 2001; 28: 7–14.

Ludwig H, Birgegard G, Olmi P et al: European Cancer Anemia Survey (ECAS): prospective evaluation of anemia in over 15,000 cancer patients [abstract]. Ann Oncol 2003; 13(Suppl): Abstract # 623.

Ludwig H, van Belle S, Barret-L P et al: The European Cancer Anaemia Survey (ECAS): a large, multinational, prospective survey defining the prevalence, incidence, and treatment of anaemia in cancer patients. Eur J Cancer 2004; 40: 2293–306.

Mercadante S, Gebbia V, Marrazzo A, Filosto S: Anaemia in cancer: pathophysiology and treatment. Cancer Treat Rev 2000; 26: 303–11.

Ortega A, Dranitsaris G, Puodziunas A: A clinical and economic evaluation of red blood cell transfusions in patients receiving cancer chemotherapy. Int J Technol Assess Health Care 1998; 14: 788–98.

Rizzo JD, Lichtin AE, Woolf SH et al: Use of epoetin in patients with cancer: evidence-based clinical practice guidelines of the American Society of Clinical Oncology and the American Society of Hematology. J Clin Oncol 2002; 20: 4083–107.

17 Febrile neutropenia

VCG Tjan-Heijnen, JNH Timmer-Bonte
Department of Medical Oncology, University Medical Centre
Nijmegen (St Radboud), the Netherlands

Introduction

Febrile neutropenia is defined as a combination of an absolute neutrophil count of less than 0.5×10^9/L (or predicted to decline below 0.5×10^9/L) and an increased temperature, i.e., an oral temperature >38.3°C (101°F), or ≥38.0°C (100.4°F) over at least 1 hour.

Febrile neutropenia should be considered as a medical emergency. The majority of patients with febrile neutropenia have occult bacterial infections despite the lack of other signs or symptoms of infection. Early studies demonstrated a nearly 70% mortality if administration of broad-spectrum intravenous antibiotics was delayed.

In cases of neutropenia without fever, an underlying infection should be considered in cases where symptoms are compatible with infection (e.g. abdominal pain), in elderly patients or patients receiving corticosteroids who have a clinical deterioration and in case of hypothermia and/or hypotension.

The incidence of febrile neutropenia increases with the severity and duration of neutropenia, the severity of mucositis throughout the gastrointestinal tract, the presence of tumor-related obstruction (e.g. lung or urinary tract) and the presence of other comorbidity.

Etiology

Infections are clinically documented in 50% of episodes of febrile neutropenia, and microbiologically in only 25%. Historically, life-threatening Gram-negative micro-organisms, particularly *Pseudomonas aeruginosa*, *Escherichia coli* and *Klebsiella* spp., were the most commonly identified pathogens.

Currently, two-thirds of microbiologically documented infections during febrile neutropenia are Gram-positive infections. Many of the Gram-positive infections are susceptible only to vancomycin and teicoplanin: coagulase-negative staphylococci (*Staphylococcus epidermidis*) are more indolent and a few days' delay in administration of specific therapy may not be detrimental. However, *Staphylococcus aureus*, viridans streptococci, penicillin-resistant *Streptococcus pneumoniae* and certain enterococci may cause fulminant infections if they are not treated immediately.

Of great concern has been the increasing frequency of antibiotic-resistant organisms. These pathogens include coagulase-negative *Staphylococcus*, methicillin-resistant *Staphylococcus aureus*, vancomycin-resistant *Enterococcus*, and penicillin-resistant *Streptococcus pneumoniae*. It is important to be aware of institutional infection and susceptibility patterns.

It is usually not necessary to add specific anaerobic antibiotic coverage to the initial empiric regimen, but this should be considered if there is evidence of necrotizing mucositis, perirectal abscess/cellulitis, intra-abdominal or pelvic infection, typhilitis (necrotizing neutropenic colitis), sinus or periodontal abscess, or anaerobic bacteremia.

Fungal pathogens (*Candida*, *Aspergillus*) usually arise later as a secondary infection in patients with prolonged neutropenia and antibiotic use.

Herpes simplex or zoster viruses are common causes of skin eruptions, and can also cause encephalitis, meningitis, myelitis, esophagitis, pneumonia, hepatitis, erythema multiforme and ocular syndromes. Other common viral infections that occur in the neutropenic host include cytomegalovirus, Epstein–Barr virus, respiratory syncytial and influenza A viruses.

Evaluation of febrile neutropenia

- Careful history.
- Register day of onset of fever to first day of last chemotherapy cycle: this permits an estimate of expected duration of neutropenia.
- It is important to remember that signs of inflammation can be extremely subtle in the neutropenic patient and even minor erythema may warrant further investigation of a site.
- Physical examination includes examination of the skin (around the nails), sinuses, fundi, oropharynx, lung, abdomen, surgical sites and perirectal area. It is important to avoid the use of a rectal thermometer in neutropenic patients. A digital rectal examination generally should also be avoided, except when a perirectal abscess or prostatitis is suspected (after broad-spectrum antibiotics have been administered).

- All indwelling lines should be carefully examined for signs of infection, erythema, tenderness, fluctuation or an exsudate that may be the only evidence of a serious "tunnel" line infection. Difficulty with infusion or blood drawing could be a sign of an infected clot even in the absence of a problem with the exit site.
- History and physical examination should be repeated daily.
- Assess complete blood counts with differential, transaminases, bilirubin, sodium, potassium and creatinine levels. Repeat these tests at least every third day and blood cell counts on a daily basis until full recovery.
- Examination of two blood cultures (some prefer culturing each intravenous port and at least one peripheral blood culture), and on indication Gram stain and culture of sputum, urine and exuding fluid of suspicious sites. Diarrhea should be tested for *Clostridium difficile* toxin, for bacteria (*Salmonella*, *Shigella*, *Campylobacter*, *Aeromonas* and *Yersinia*), viruses (Rotavirus or Cytomegalovirus) or protozoa (*Cryptosporidium* spp).
- Blood cultures should be repeated for persistent fevers or rigors once a day or, alternatively, repeated 48–72 hours after initial cultures unless the patient has hemodynamic instability, rigors, new localizing symptoms or another clinical change. Lumbar puncture is not usually recommended but should be considered if symptoms are suggestive of a central nervous system (CNS) infection.
- At presentation, chest X-ray should always be performed, and repeated for persistent pulmonary symptoms. Chest X-ray findings are often minimal or absent even in patients with pneumonia, until neutropenia begins to resolve. Other imaging techniques (ultrasonography, CT scan, MRI scan) should be considered in those with persistent fever or signs of infection.
- Perform risk assessment to identify patients at risk for serious complications (one of the following factors present):
  - in-patient at presentation
  - significant co-morbidity
  - clinical instability or complex infections such as pneumonia
  - abnormal renal or liver function
  - progressive tumor
  - stem cell transplantation recipients
  - anticipated severe (<100/µL) neutropenia of more than 7 days
  - Multinational Association of Supportive Care in Cancer (MASCC) score of 21 or less (Table 17.1).

Table 17.1 MASSC score

Characteristic	Weight
Burden of illness:	
no symptoms or mild symptoms	5
moderate symptoms	3
No hypotension	5
No chronic obstructive pulmonary disease	4
Solid tumor or hematological malignancy with fungal infection	4
No dehydration	3
Out-patient status	3
Age <60 years old	2

Treatment of febrile neutropenia

- Administer broad-spectrum bactericidal antibiotics promptly by the intravenous route and in maximal therapeutic dosage.
- Check for drug allergy or organ dysfunction (especially renal).
- Combinations of nephrotoxic drugs such as (recent) cisplatin, cyclosporine, amphotericin B and aminoglycosides should be avoided.
- Drug plasma concentrations of aminoglycosides should be monitored.
- Catheter-related infections:
  - routine use of urokinase is not recommended.
  - administration of antibiotics alternating through each lumen is recommended.
  - do not remove catheter if catheter-related bacteremia or entry-site infection.
  - catheter should be removed if positive blood culture with fungi or mycobacteria, response to antibiotics delayed >48 hours, tunnel infection, septic emboli, hypotension or non-patent catheter.

Initial treatment of febrile neutropenia

Check local susceptibility patterns.

- Indications for vancomycin:
  - severe mucositis
  - quinolone prophylaxis

- colonization with resistant microorganisms
- institutions where fulminant Gram-positive bacterial infections are common
- obvious catheter-related infection
- hypotension
- positive blood culture for Gram-positive bacteria before final identification: vancomycin + antipseudomonal beta-lactam (ceftazidime).

■ No indication for vancomycin:
- monotherapy – ceftazidim or imipenem
- duotherapy – aminoglycoside + antipseudomonal beta-lactam.

These drugs do not usually provide coverage for coagulase-negative staphylococci, methicillin-resistant *Staphylococcus aureus*, enterococci, some strains of penicillin-resistant *Streptococcus pneumoniae*, and viridans streptococci.

■ Reassess after 3 days.

Afebrile within first 3 days of treatment

■ Etiology identified: adjust to most appropriate treatment, but also keep broad-spectrum coverage in case of persistent neutropenia.
■ Etiology not identified:
- high risk – continue same antibiotics
- low risk – change to oral antibiotics (cefixime or quinolone) + discharge.
■ Duration of antibiotic therapy:
- if early bone marrow recovery, stop antibiotics when 2 days without fever and absolute neutrophil count $\geq 0.5 \times 10^9$/L
- stop antibiotics after 7 days when absolute neutrophil count $\geq 0.5 \times 10^9$/L by day 7
- when absolute neutrophil count $< 0.5 \times 10^9$/L by day 7 –
  (1) high risk, continue antibiotics; (2) low risk and clinically well, stop when 5–7 days without fever.

Persistent fever during first 3 days of treatment without etiology

Reassess on days 4–5: presence of non-bacterial infection, a resistant bacterial infection (note that it may require 4–5 days of therapy before defervescence occurs), emergence of second infection, inadequate tissue levels of antibiotics, drug fever, infection at vascular site (abscesses or catheters):

- Continue initial antibiotics (if no change, consider stopping vancomycin).
- Change or add antibiotics (repeated cultures):
  - Add vancomycin to Gram-negative coverage based on cultures or because of life-threatening sepsis.
  - Add amphotericin B with or without changing antibiotics if fever persists through days 5–7 and resolution of neutropenia is not imminent. Every effort should be made to first determine whether or not systemic fungal infection exists. Fluconazole may be an acceptable alternative.
- Duration of antibiotic therapy with persistent fever:
  - Absolute neutrophil count $\geq 0.5 \times 10^9$/L: stop 4–5 days after absolute neutrophil count recovery and reassess.
  - Absolute neutrophil count $<0.5 \times 10^9$/L: continue 2 weeks, reassess, stop if no disease sites and stable clinical situation.
- Use of antiviral drugs only in case of evidence of viral infections:
  - Herpes simplex or varicella-zoster virus: acyclovir.
  - Cytomegalovirus: ganciclovir or foscarnet.
  - Respiratory syncytial virus: ribavirin.
  - Influenza A: rimantadine or amantadine.

Granulocyte colony-stimulating factor

For the majority of patients with febrile neutropenia, there is no clear support for the routine initiation of granulocyte colony-stimulating factors as adjuncts to antibiotic therapy. However, certain patients may have prognostic factors that are predictive of clinical deterioration, such as pneumonia, hypotension, multiorgan dysfunction (sepsis syndrome), or fungal infection. The use of CSFs together with antibiotics may be reasonable in such high-risk patients.

- Primary granulocyte colony-stimulating factor prophylaxis to prevent febrile neutropenia is generally not recommended for standard dose chemotherapy, except for patients who have potential risk factors for febrile neutropenia or infection.
- Secondary granulocyte-colony stimulating factor prophylaxis after an episode of febrile neutropenia should be considered in curable tumors. Alternatives for secondary prophylaxis are dose reductions of chemotherapy or use of prophylactic antibiotics.

Future directions

There is a growing interest in identifying low-risk patients and the use of (oral) antimicrobial therapy on an outpatient basis, but these approaches cannot be adopted yet, although first study results are encouraging.

Further reading

Hughes WT, Armstrong D, Bodey GP, et al: Guidelines for the use of antimicrobial agents in neutropenic patients with unexplained fever. Clin Infect Dis 1997; 25: 551–73.

Ozer H, Armitage JO, Bennett CL et al for the ASCO Growth Factors Expert Panel: 2000 update of recommendations for the use of hematopoietic colony-stimulating factors: evidence-based, clinical practice guidelines. J Clin Oncol 2000; 18: 3558–85.

Bleeding disorders

18

K De Leeuw, D Schrijvers
Ziekenhuisnetwerk-Middelheim, Belgium

Introduction

Bleeding complications in cancer patients may be due to cancer or to anti-cancer treatment; they may be life-threatening and should be adequately recognized and treated.

Overall, the most common cause of hemorrhage in cancer patients is thrombocytopenia (50%). Thrombocytopenia may be the result of treatment with chemotherapy or bone marrow involvement by cancer, but it can also be caused by consumptive coagulopathy, immune-mediated mechanisms, infection or sequestration.

In patients with solid tumors and treated with chemotherapy, bleeding due to thrombocytopenia is seen in 9–15%. Cancer patients with similar depth and duration of thrombocytopenia share a common risk of bleeding, regardless of the chemotherapy regimen that is administered.

Severe hemorrhage is uncommon with platelet counts higher than 10 000/µl to 20 000/µl or with slowly decreasing platelet counts.

Risk factors for a chemotherapy-induced thrombocytopenia and bleeding are a history of bleeding; poor bone marrow function with a low baseline platelet count; bone marrow metastases; and poor performance status.

When bleeding occurs in patients with chemotherapy-induced thrombocytopenia, it is associated with poor clinical outcomes and significantly increased resource utilization.

Etiology

The hemostatic system can be significantly altered by cancer and its treatment. There may be interference with the clotting system, the platelet number and function and the vessel wall. The main causes of bleeding are given in Table 18.1.

Table 18.1 Causes of bleeding in cancer patients

System	Syndrome	Occurrence
Clotting system	Decreased clotting factors; coagulation factor abnormalities	Liver disease
		Cholestasis
		Drug-induced
		Acquired von Willebrand's disease
	Disseminated intravascular clotting	Leukemia cell procoagulant activity
		Bacteremia
		Massive transfusion
		Shock
	Primary fibrinolysis; fibrinogenolysis	Leukemia cell proteolytic activity
		Drug-induced
	Circulatory anticoagulants	Factor inhibitors
		Heparin-like anticoagulants
Thrombocytes	Thrombocytopenia	Immune thrombocytopenia
		Bone marrow infiltration
		Drug-induced
	Platelet dysfunction	Myeloproliferative syndromes
		Acute leukemia
		Preleukemia
		Hairy-cell leukemia
		Drug-induced
Vessels	Vascular defects	Infiltration
		Hyperviscosity/leukostasis
		Extramedullary hematopoiesis

Clotting system

Decreased production of clotting factors

■ Liver involvement by cancer can cause defective or decreased synthesis of coagulation factors II, VII, IX, X, XI, XII, XIII, prekallikrein, high-molecular-weight kininogen, plasminogen, antithrombin III, protein S and protein C.

- Acquired von Willebrand's disease is seen in association with hematologic malignancies.
- Drug-induced: coumarin derivates, cephalosporins, asparaginase.

Fibrinolysis

- Primary fibrinolysis due to local or systemic activation of the fibrinolytic system, resulting in plasmin degradation of fibrin, fibrinogen, factor V and factor VIII is observed in patients with sarcomas, breast, thyroid, colon and stomach cancer and hematologic malignancies.
- Secondary fibrinolysis due to diffuse intravascular coagulation (DIC).
- Solid tumors are capable of inducing fibrinolytic activity.

Thrombocytes

Thrombocytopenia

- Impaired production due to chemotherapy or radiotherapy.
- Splenic sequestration in patients with splenomegaly.
- Immune-mediated thrombocytopenia related to anti-HLA, paraproteins or antiplatelet-specific alloantibodies may be seen in chronic lymphocytic leukemia, non-Hodgkin's lymphoma, Hodgkin's disease, lung, breast and gastrointestinal cancer.
- Diffuse intravascular coagulation is associated with acute myelocytic leukemia, lymphoma and carcinoma of lung, breast, gastrointestinal or urologic origin. DIC most commonly complicates acute promyelocytic leukemia due to the presence of both thromboplastic material and fibrinolytic proteases in the promyelocytic subcellular components.

Abnormal platelet function

- Chronic myeloproliferative disorders with decreased platelet procoagulant activity and decreased aggregation and serotonin release responses to adenosine diphophate (ADP), epinephrine (adrenaline) or collagen.
- Paraproteins may impair platelet aggregation (IgA myeloma, Waldenström's macroglobulinemia, multiple myeloma, monoclonal gammopathy of undetermined significance).
- Thrombocytosis: platelet dysfunction can be associated with elevated platelet counts (greater than $700\,000/\mu l$)
- Hyperviscosity.
- Acquired factor X deficiency in the setting of amyloidosis.
- Circulating heparin-like anticoagulant.

■ Drug-induced: heparin, low-molecular-weight heparin, nonsteroidal anti-inflammatory drugs (NSAIDs), beta-lactams, amphotericin B, plicamycin, vincristine, nitrofurantoin.

Evaluation

Symptoms

Depending on the extent and location of bleeding, patients may complain of palpitation, fatigue, dyspnea, hematuria, epistaxis, headache or visual disturbances.

Clinical examination

Localized bleeding should be determined by clinical examination:

■ mucosal bleeding with gingival bleeding
■ skin lesions with spontaneous bruising, petechiae, purpura
■ bleeding from the sites of indwelling catheters or puncture sites
■ bleeding at pulmonary, central nervous system (CNS), gastrointestinal or genitourinary sites.

Laboratory examinations

Hematologic evaluation

■ Cytology: number and differentiation of white blood cells; number of platelets.
■ Blood film examination: schistocytes in DIC.
■ Platelet function tests comprise platelet function closure time and bleeding time.

Coagulation parameters

■ Activated partial thromboplastin time (aPTT) measures intrinsic pathway and is prolonged by factor VIII and IX deficiency.
■ Prothrombin time (PT) measures extrinsic pathway.
■ Both aPPT and PT are affected by factor X, factor V, prothrombin and fibrinogen.
■ Thrombin time measures common pathway.
■ Fibrinogen and fibrinogen degradation products (D-dimers).
■ Von Willebrand's factor.
■ Coomb's test.
■ Autoimmune thrombocytopenia in association with autoimmune hemolytic anemia gives a positive antiglobulin test.

Biochemical analyses

◼ Urea, creatinine, liver function tests and protein electrophoresis.

Bone marrow examination

◼ In case of suspicion of immune-mediated thrombocytopenia.
◼ Suspicion of plasma cell proliferation.

Echo abdomen

◼ To detect splenomegaly and liver metastases.

Prevention and treatment

Prevention of bleeding

Chemotherapy-induced thrombocytopenia

◼ If platelets <10 000/µl: platelet transfusion infusions of 6–8 units every 1–2 days until platelet counts remain above 10 000/µl.
◼ For invasive procedures: platelets >30 000/µl.
◼ For surgery: platelets >50 000/µl (Table 18.2).

Coagulation

◼ Antibiotic therapy: monitoring of PT and aPTT.
◼ Heparin therapy: monitoring of aPTT.
◼ Vitamin K antagonists: monitoring of international normalized ratio (INR).

Table 18.2 Indications for platelet transfusions

Trigger (platelets/µl)	Clinical status
<10 000	Stable, absence of active bleeding
10 000–20 000	Presence of coagulation disorders
	Infection with fever >38°C (and rapid decrease of platelets)
	Local injuries
	Severe mucositis, active bleeding
	Biopsy (except bone marrow biopsy)
<50 000	Surgery

Treatment of bleeding
Chemotherapy-induced thrombocytopenia

Platelet transfusion until platelets >30 000/µl.

- Only products that are leukocyte-reduced (either by filtration or by irradiation) should be given to avoid early alloimmunization.
- Transfusion of 4–6 pooled random donor platelet concentrates is normally as effective as single-donor apheresis products, depending on the content of platelets and the duration of storage of each product.
- Platelets should be given as random ABO-compatible (non-HLA-typed) transfusions.
- HLA-matched transfusions or cross-matched platelets should only be given in patients refractory to at least 2 random platelet transfusions.
- The effectiveness of platelet transfusion can be assessed by the corrected increment (increment in platelet counts from before to after transfusion corrected for the number of units transfused and for the body surface area of the recipient) in platelet count 1 hour or the bleeding time 10–15 minutes after transfusion and the observed clinical outcome after transfusion.

Thrombocytosis

Platelet dysfunction associated with elevated platelet counts (greater than 700 000/µl) can be corrected by platelet apheresis.

Platelet dysfunction

Platelet dysfunction due to paraproteinemia can be treated with plasma apheresis.

Coagulation disturbances
Liver disease

Bleeding due to liver disease causing defective or decreased synthesis of coagulation factors II, VII, IX, X, XI, XII, XIII, prekallikrein, high-molecular-weight kininogen, plasminogen, antithrombin III, protein S and protein C can be corrected by replacement of vitamin K or the appropriate coagulation factors.

Acquired von Willebrand's disease

- Infusion of cryoprecipitate: factor VIII and von Willebrand's factor in a dose of 25 IU/kg with as target a factor VIII level of more than 30% of normal level until bleeding stops (usually 2–4 days)
- Desmopressin administered at a dose of 0.3 μg per kilogram of body weight by continuous intravenous infusion for 30 minutes.

Fibrinolysis

- Tranexamic acid 500 mg every 8–12 hours orally or intravenously.
- Epsilon-aminocaproic acid 5–10 g slow intravenous loading dose followed by 1–2 g/h for 24 hours followed by oral administration (Figure 18.1).

Diffuse intravascular coagulation

- Observation in patients who are not bleeding and platelet count more than 10 000/μl and no coagulopathy.
- Platelet transfusion if platelet count is less than 10 000/μl.
- Coagulopathy: fresh frozen plasma, fibrinogen concentrate or cryoprecipitate.

Local bleeding

Local bleeding should be controlled by local measurements.

- In case of visible bleeding, pressure may stop bleeding if the clotting system is intact.
- Heat (laser) coagulation may be used in local treatment of gastrointestinal bleeding.
- Arterial embolization by angiography may be used to stop arterial bleeding in different organ systems.
- Surgical intervention may be necessary to control local bleeding.
- Radiotherapy may be used to give a hemostatic radiation in case of urogenital or pulmonary bleeding.

Conclusion

Bleeding is a life-threatening condition in cancer patients. Prevention and treatment should be integrated in chemotherapy protocols.

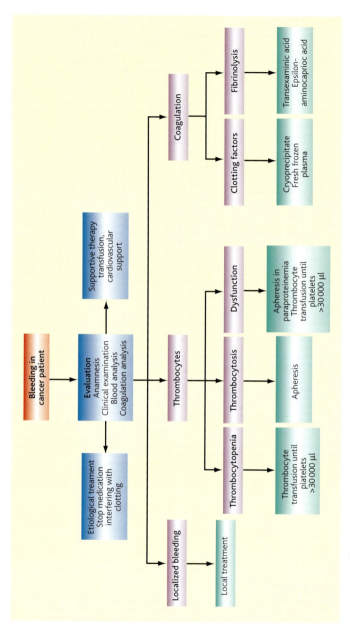

Figure 18.1 Algorithm of bleeding in the cancer patient.

Further reading

Elting LE, Rubenstein EB, Martin CG et al: Incidence, cost, and outcomes of bleeding and chemotherapy dose modification among solid tumor patients with chemotherapy-induced thrombocytopenia. J Clin Oncol 2001; 19: 1137–46.

Mannucci PM: Treatment of von Willebrand's disease. N Engl J Med 2004; 351: 683–94.

Schiffer CA, Anderson KC, Bennett CL et al: Platelet transfusion for patients with cancer: clinical practice guidelines of the American Society of Clinical Oncology. J Clin Oncol 2001; 19: 1519–38.

Wandt H, Ehninger G, Gallmeier WM: New strategies for prophylactic platelet transfusion in patients with hematologic diseases. Oncologist 2001; 6: 446–50.

19 Management of cancer pain

M Di Palma
Institut Gustave Roussy, France

Introduction

Pain is one of the most dreaded symptoms of cancer: at diagnosis, 50% of patients suffer pain; during treatment, 30% of patients have pain; and at the end of their life, 90% of patients are experiencing pain.

Etiology

The etiology of cancer pain is given in Box 19.1.

Evaluation

Anamnesis of cancer pain

When a cancer patient is referred for a cancer pain, the first step consists of defining cancer pain. Cancer pain will be defined and classified according to five criteria.

Type of cancer pain

According to the pathophysiology:

- Nociceptive pain due to stimulation of nociceptors:
    - somatic cancer pain
    - visceral cancer pain.
- Neuropathic cancer pain: damage to nerve tissue.

Temporal aspects of cancer pain

- Acute pain is a pain with a well-defined temporal pattern of pain onset.
- Chronic pain is usually defined as the persistence of pain for more than 3 months, with a less defined temporal onset.

Box 19.1 Causes of pain in cancer patients

Tumor invasion (70%):
- Bone invasion
- Obstruction of hollow organ or duct system
- Mucous membrane ulceration
- Obstruction or invasion of vascular structures
- Compression or invasion of neural structures

Diagnosis and treatment (20%):
- Diagnostic and staging procedures
- Surgery
- Radiotherapy (e.g., mucositis, enteritis, neurotoxicity)
- Chemotherapy (e.g., mucositis, neurotoxicity)

Cancer-induced syndromes (< 10%):
- Debility (constipation, rectal or bladder spasm)
- Paraneoplastic syndromes

Unrelated to cancer or cancer treatment:
- Cardiac infarction
- Ischemic disease
- Other

Intensity and measurements

The intensity should be evaluated with one of the following tools:

- visual analog scale
- brief pain inventory
- McGill pain questionnaire
- memorial pain assessment card.

Previous and ongoing treatment

Any previous analgesic treatment should be assessed.

Etiology

Cancer pain may also be classified as tumor-related or treatment-related. This classification is of importance when considering treatment.

Clinical examination

A careful clinical examination should be performed to detect the cause of the pain.

Technical examinations

Technical examinations should be reserved for when there is doubt to the cause of pain or when it influences treatment:

- plain radiographs may be used as screening
- a computed tomography (CT) scan to evaluate bone, soft tissue structures and organs (brain)
- a magnetic resonance image (MRI) to evaluate the spine
- echography/doppler echography
- radioisotopes in case of bone metastases.

Treatment

Classes of drugs

Nonopioid analgesics

This class includes aspirin, nonsteroidal anti-inflammatory drugs (NSAIDs) and acetaminophen (paracetamol).

These drugs are usually given to patients with low to moderate pain as step 1 analgesics (World Health Organization (WHO) classification). They can be associated with opioid drugs.

Opioid analgesics

This class includes step 2 and step 3 analgesics (WHO classification):

- Step 2 includes weak opioids: e.g., codeine, propoxyphene or tramadol.
- Step 3 includes strong opioids: e.g., morphine, fentanyl or hydromorphone.

Adjuvants analgesics

- Tricyclic antidepressant drugs: amitriptyline, clomipramine or imipramine.
- Anticonvulsant drugs: gabapentin, carbamazepine.
- Corticosteroids.
- Bisphosphonates.
- Muscle relaxing drugs: butylhyoscine, benzodiazopines.

Principles of treatment

Appropriate drug for a specific situation

Nociceptive pain

Step 1/2 or 3 of the WHO pain ladder, according to the intensity.

Example:

Morphine intravenous or subcutaneously: 10–20 mg every 4 hours with escape of 10 mg; calculate daily dose needed for pain control and change to other route of administraton (equianalgesic dose)

Morphine orally: 10–20 mg every 4 hours with escape of 10 mg, calculate daily dose needed for pain control and change to SR morphine (dose is same as of daily dose of immediate acting morphine),

Practical considerations

In the context of emergency, avoid morphine with long half-life (requires 6–24 hours to be active). Only physicians familiar with opioids should titrate morphine. In other situations, start treatment by conventional dose of morphine (compare with above). Surveillance of vital emergency is necessary and naloxone (antidote) must be available. Example of protocol for titration: morphine 2 mg intravenously/5 minutes until disappearance of pain.

Neuropathic pain

Opioids are usually not efficient in this type of pain, but should be tried.

Tricyclic antidepressants or anticonvulsants should be used.

Example

Amitriptyline: 10–25 mg/day starting dose, and titrate up to achieve analgesia.

Gabapentin: 300 mg/day starting dose; then titrate up to achieve analgesia. The dose is usually between 900 and 1800 mg/day.

Appropriate doses + knowledge of equivalence

The oral starting dose of morphine is 60 mg/day in patients with severe pain. It is necessary to know the different equivalent doses of the different drugs (Table 19.1).

Table 19.1 *Equianalgesic doses and activity of opioids*

Opioid	Route of administration	Equianalgesic dose	Activity (hours)
Morphine	Oral	30 mg	4
	Subcutaneous	10 mg	4
	Intravenous	10 mg	4
SR morphine	Oral	30 mg	12–24
SR hydromorphone	Oral	4 mg	12–24
Fentanyl patch	Transcutaneous	8 µg	72
Buprenorphine patch	Transcutaneous	16 µg	72

Appropriate route of administration

Most analgesics are given orally. However, opioids may also be given subcutaneously or intravenously. In specific situations they may be given intrathecally.

There are patches available to administer opioids transcutaneously. These should not be used to treat acute pain. Once the pain is controlled they may be started with an overlap with the short-acting opioid.

By the clock

Analgesics should be taken on fixed hours to prevent pain. In addition, escape medication should be prescribed.

The transcutaneous patches may facilitate the continuous administration of opioids.

Use of adjuvant treatment if necessary

- Bone metastases: corticosteroids, bisphosphonates.
- Tumor-related headache (edema): corticosteroids.
- Visceral dilatation: antispasmodics.
- Muscle spasm: benzodiazepines.
- Other treatment modalities:
  - radiotherapy
  - neurologic blocks.

Anticipate and treat side effects

- Use antiemetics and laxatives with opioids.
- Start with a lower dose in elderly patients (e.g., 50% of normal dose).
- Be aware of anticholinergic effect of tricyclic antidepressants.
- Opioid rotation: if a specific opioid causes too many side effects, change to another opioid:
  - calculate equianalgesic dose
  - decrease equianalgesic dose by 25–50%, except for fentanyl
  - rescue dose is 5–10% of total daily dose.
- Treat etiology if possible.
- Special situations:
  - Patients with pre-existing treatment who present with acute pain: in this subset of patients, the most crucial point is to understand the reason why the pain is not controlled by treatment.
    - For *a new cause of pain*: treat the new cause with the appropriate drug + etiology.
    - For *a progressive disease*: (1) adapt according to the WHO pain ladder; (2) increase the dose of the drug by 50–100%; and (3) add a new drug.

Opioid overdose

Opioid overdosage is characterized by sedation and respiratory depression. When such a clinical situation is detected, the presence of myosis (pinpoint pupils) is a useful sign to diagnose a morphine overdose.

Naloxone is the antagonist of opioids. It is administered intravenously in a dose of 0.1 mg every 2–3 minutes, until a dose of 0.4–2 mg is reached.

Sedation is usually not an indication for naloxone if the patient can be awakened, and if there is no respiratory depression.

In case the of fever, transdermal fentanyl should be used with caution, since the risk of overdosage is increased due to increased resorption.

Pain related to visceral obstruction

Pain related to visceral dilatation should be treated with antispasmodics.

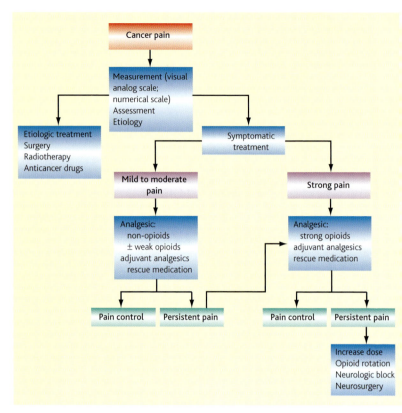

Figure 19.1 Algorithm for pain management

Further reading

Cherny NI, Chang V, Frager G et al: Opioid pharmacotherapy in the management of cancer pain. Cancer 1995; 76: 1283.

Donnelly S, Davis MP, Walsh D, Naughton M: World Health Organization. Morphine in cancer pain management: a practical guide. Support Care Cancer 2002; 10: 13–35.

Foley K: Management of cancer pain. In: De Vita VT Jr, Hellman S, Rosenburg SA (eds), Cancer: Principles and Practice of Oncology, 6th edn. Philadelphia: Lippincott-Raven, 2002: 2977–3012.

Gourlay GK: Treatment of cancer pain with transdermal fentanyl. Lancet Oncol 2001; 2: 165–72.

World Health Organization. Cancer Pain Relief, 2nd edn. Geneva: World Health Organization, 1996.

Index